TREATMENT OF CEREBRAL PALSY
AND MOTOR DELAY

TREATMENT OF CEREBRAL PALSY AND MOTOR DELAY

SOPHIE LEVITT

BSc (Physiotherapy) Rand.

Supervisor of Therapy Studies
Wolfson Centre
Institute of Child Health
London

With a foreword by
MARY D. SHERIDAN
MA MD DCH

BLACKWELL SCIENTIFIC PUBLICATIONS

OXFORD LONDON EDINBURGH MELBOURNE

© 1977 Blackwell Scientific Publications
Editorial offices:
Osney Mead, Oxford OX2 0EL
8 John Street, London WC1N 2ES
9 Forrest Road, Edinburgh EH1 2QH
214 Berkeley Street, Carlton, Victoria 3053, Australia.

First published 1977
Reprinted 1979

British Library Cataloguing in Publication Data

Levitt, Sophie
Treatment of cerebral palsy and motor delay.
1. Cerebral palsied children
I. Title
618.9′28′3606   RJ496.C4

ISBN 0–632–00931–4

DISTRIBUTORS

USA
    Blackwell Mosby Book Distributors
    11830 Westline Industrial Drive
    St Louis, Missouri 63141

Canada
    Blackwell Mosby Book Distributors
    86 Northline Road, Toronto
    Ontario, M4B 3E5

Australia
    Blackwell Scientific Book
    Distributors
    214 Berkeley Street, Carlton
    Victoria 3053

Set in Century Schoolbook
Printed and bound in Great Britain
at the Alden Press, Oxford.

CONTENTS

FOREWORD

The happy accident of being a fellow lecturer on a course in developmental paediatrics some years ago brought about my first introduction to Sophie Levitt's work. My attention was immediately engaged by the gentle but firm authority with which she expounded her message to us, an experienced professional audience, and by her well-chosen lantern slides. Later I was impressed by her ease in rapidly establishing good relationships with half a dozen young handicapped children and their mothers who had been called for demonstration, and were previously unknown to her; but above all the lovely competence of her 'laying on of hands' filled me with admiration. Since then I have welcomed any opportunity open to me to see and listen to her in action. No greater compliment than this can be paid by one teacher to another.

She tells us that her aim has been to concentrate on the mechanisms of posture, balance, locomotion and manipulation in normal and physically abnormal children. She discusses how these mechanisms occur, how they are maintained, and how they must be trained to ensure optimum development of mobility and hand skills. But her book covers much wider ground. Experience has taught her the importance of a host of other influences which must be taken into serious consideration in treatment of a child and the counselling of parents. She stresses the importance of a comprehensive assessment which is not mere 'reflex hunting' but takes into account a child's present levels of visual, auditory and language development, his intelligence and personality, and, very importantly the prognosis of his disability. She points out the parents' needs for consistent sympathetic knowledgeable guidance and the necessity for adequate local services for follow-up supervision and education.

Whilst the largest part of her book is devoted to description of, and detailed explanation of, the principles underlying her own therapeutic procedures which she has evolved from wide clinical experience and the selection of some acknowledgeably successful items from numerous previous 'systems', she also provides much helpful advice on other aspects of treatment and training.

The photographs are clear and well-chosen. The drawings are a sheer delight. The book cannot fail to inform and inspire many other workers in the field of developmental paediatrics as it has informed, inspired and indeed comforted me.

Mary D. Sheridan

PREFACE

'What makes a child move?' is a crucial question for those treating cerebral palsied children and children with developmental motor delay. Various answers to this question come from different doctors, physiotherapists, occupational therapists as well as from psychologists and educationalists. In addition those disciplines concerned with deprived social and economic conditions and with the design of environments for handicapped children will offer reasons for limitation of children's movement development through lack of stimulation and motor exploration.

Although recognising the value of all these ideas, this book is based on the answers given by different doctors, therapists and my own experience. Many workers in this field, in various countries, have generously given me of their time and knowledge. Space does not permit mention of all their names, but they have my deep gratitude. I am particularly appreciative of the privilege of discussions and observations of the work of Dr Phelps, Dr and Mrs Bobath, Dr Fay, Dr Vojta, Miss Knott, Mrs Collis and Dr Hari. They have inspired and influenced me and without them this book could not have been written. Although I have been emotionally drawn to follow each one of them devotedly out of respect for their great contributions, I could not do so. It would have been a denial of my own thoughts and experience, and I hope they will respect this. I have dared to stand on their broad shoulders and attempt to synthesise some of their ideas at this stage of our knowledge.

In working out this synthesis, it has been especially helpful and stimulating to work for many years with Dr John Foley and benefit from his studies and interpretations of J. Purdon Martin's work in adult and child neurology. I have been encouraged in my eclectic viewpoint not only by Dr Foley and the staff of the Cheyne Walk Spastic Centre, but also by my present Director, Professor Kenneth Holt, and by the late Professor Robert Collis, by Professor G. Tardieu and many students and colleagues.

My attempts to correlate the neurology of Foley and Purdon Martin to child development depended on the extensive use of the work of Dr Mary Sheridan. She is an inspiration to me and many of my colleagues. It is a special honour to have a Foreword by her. I am most grateful.

My experience is also greatly dependent on the parents and children with whom I have been privileged to work and learn so much. It is because of their essential participation that I was unable to write a book 'for therapists only' and the large section on practical procedures (Chapter 6)

is divided into *Treatment suggestions* which can be carried out by both
therapists and parents under *Daily care*. These methods must, however, be
selected for the child by a physiotherapist and then *shown* to the parents,
or to surrogate parents such as nursery nurses, teachers, playgroup workers
and others. The others also include speech therapists and occupational
therapists who offer their methods to the physiotherapist when indicated.
The book includes some of their suggestions.

Parents and therapists
This book takes special account of parents as their cooperation is needed
to correctly handle their child throughout the day, sometimes carry out
special exercises or manipulations, apply any calipers and use the special
aids, correct toys, footwear and other recommendations of therapists.
This book, however, does not elaborate on the attitudes of parents which
affect the use of the many practical ideas offered. Parents' attitudes are
known to affect the progress of their handicapped child. The subject is a
vast one as parents are people and the variety of attitudes among people
requires much discussion. Many other books have been written on the
subject and should be consulted. It is however, the day-to-day experience of
communicating with parents and the advice of various other disciplines
working with these parents that will educate the therapist. She must also
observe what she does to influence parents' attitudes negatively as well as
positively. In summary, the therapist must learn:

    To communicate TO parents why methods are selected and further
explain or repeat what the doctors have said about the child's problems.
She must instruct parents in how to do the methods and give them confidence in doing them. She must then have an ongoing supervision of these
methods which should be primarily those concerned with the child's daily
activities.

    To receive communication FROM parents as to their practical problems
and needs, their own suggestions and discoveries, their observations of
their child and the questions they really want answered. Receiving communication from parents and the team of workers will also help the therapist
put her treatment in a context which is relevant to the child AND his
parents and family. This takes skill so that the parents do not exaggerate
their role as 'therapists' to the detriment of the family. Treatment of the
handicapped child should not create a handicapped family under severe
strain.

The plan of the book
The aim is to present as practical a book as possible as there are already
books which review systems of treatment and recommend an open mind,
but do not tell the therapist how to DO it. It is difficult to describe methods
without demonstration. Thus, the therapist should use this book with
practical courses, further study, observations and supervision by senior
colleagues.

Methods are not in themselves all important. The therapist must know the purpose of each method and if she detects the principle behind it she can invent her own methods besides those suggested in this book. Wherever possible the principle has been given, as to why, when and when not to use methods, but not all possibilities can be covered in a book. Once again, clinical experience and courses are recommended to supplement this book.

The methods have been linked with the problems of the child and rather less with the diagnosis. The causes and the disorders underlying the problem of function are of less concern to therapists and parents and are not given as much prominence in this book. It is the developmental disabilities of motor delay and motor dysfunction which are the problems. These functions are our chief concern. Dr R. MacKeith has said 'we must separate disorder from function' using disorder to mean the underlying signs and symptoms requiring diagnostic procedures.

Theory and practice is therefore presented as follows: Chapters 1 to 4 cover general and specific principles of treatment and daily care with discussion of how to synthesise the different viewpoints; Chapters 5 to 7 cover practical assessment and procedures based on this assessment. Chapter 8 presents ideas and methods from a synthesis of neurology and orthopaedics relevant to therapy. Finally, Chapter 9 applies the ideas and methods in a group situation for children. Mother-and-baby groups are not discussed as they should be observed for understanding and practice.

Swimming, horse riding, skiing and other recreational activities for the handicapped child are omitted as they are not strictly 'treatment'. They are naturally highly recommended and other publications and films are available in many countries.

It is hoped that this book will respond to some extent to the remarks of my post-graduate students and colleagues who suggested I write it. Remarks such as:

'I agree with your eclectic approach, but how do I go about doing it'.

'How is it possible to combine such different viewpoints in our field?'

'I have followed one system but would like to extend my repertoire of methods'.

'I believe in one system, but am open to hearing other viewpoints'. but especially to the remark:

'Help me help these children and their families'.

Sophie Levitt
London 1977

ACKNOWLEDGEMENTS

I am grateful to the Leverhulme Trust Fund who kindly awarded me a Research Fellowship for part of my studies on the Synthesis of Treatment Systems in Cerebral Palsy which form the foundation of this book.

This book was commenced when I was Director of Studies at the Centre for Spastic Children, Cheyne Walk, and the Centre gave me encouraging support for which I thank them.

Acknowledgement is also made for the kind and generous help of the following:

Alison Wisbeach O.T.R. for the drawings.
The Richard Cloudsley School, London EC1, especially Ted Remington, Assistant Head, for taking most of the photographs in this book, and also Christine White, Superintendent Physiotherapist, Miss Suckling, Headmistress, and her staff for all their assistance; Centre for Spastic Children, Cheyne Walk, for Figures 6.69, 6.127, 6.128, 7.3, 9.1; The Wolfson Centre and Professor K. Holt for Figures 6.11, 6.163, 6.166; Westhill Hospital, Occupational Therapy Department, in Dartford Kent for the picture of their Standing Frame in the Appendix; Forest Town School for Spastics in South Africa for photographs from my first book in Figures 6.162, 6.167; Ivan Hume for photographs in Figures 6.66, 6.67, 6.196, 6.197, 6.198, 6.199; my patient, critical and helpful readers of the manuscript who include my late husband Jack Halpern; Dr Peter Woolf, Consultant Psychiatrist; Dr Richard Lovell, Physicist, and various therapy colleagues; Dianna Wrathall as well as Jacky Deunette, Glen Smerdan and others for typing; the children who cooperated so amazingly with the long sessions of photography and to their parents as well as to all the children and parents I have been privileged to treat and work with in the past and present.

My publishers have been particularly kind, helpful and sensitive and I thank Mr P. Saugman, Mr R. Lomax and Ms C. Swales. Dr Mary Sheridan has been wonderfully encouraging and I am most grateful for her Foreword.

A special thanks to my child, David Halpern, for his patience, understanding and the numerous cups of coffee.

CHAPTER 1

PRINCIPLES OF TREATMENT

THE CLINICAL PICTURE IN CEREBRAL PALSY

This chapter does not present the *medical aspects* in isolation, but outlines the clinical picture in such a way as to make it immediately relevant to the formulation of principles of treatment.

Cerebral palsy is the commonly used name for a *group* of conditions characterised by motor dysfunction due to non-progressive brain damage early in life. One could regard the cerebral palsies as part of a continuum of dysfunction which at one end merges into the field of mental subnormality and at the other end into that of 'minimal brain dysfunction'. It is at this latter end that we find the clumsy children who are intelligent but have specific learning problems.

THE MOTOR DYSFUNCTION

The therapist should beware of a tendency to look upon the various motor disorders only as problems of stiff or weak muscles or deformed joints. For whilst it is true that in particular cases the mechanical problems posed by these abnormalities have to be treated with orthopaedic and therapy procedures, this is but a small part of treatment as a whole. The muscle and joint pictures encountered in the cerebral palsies arise from a lack of coordinating influences from the brain. In other words the neurological mechanisms of posture, balance and movement are disorganised. Therefore the muscles which are activated for maintaining posture, balance and movement, become uncoordinated or weak. The therapist should thus aim treatment primarily at the neurological mechanisms in the central nervous system which activate and control the muscles.

Unfortunately, not all the neurological mechanisms, nor the integration of neurology and psychology which account for the abnormal motor behaviour are fully understood as yet. However, sufficient neurological and psychological mechanisms are understood to serve as a practical and rational basis for treating children.

In the past the principles of treatment of many cerebral palsy therapists have largely centred on the spasticity, rigidity or athetosis, especially in relation to voluntary movements. It is, of course, necessary to pay attention to these symptoms at all times. It is, however, more important to concentrate on the mechanisms of posture, balance and locomotion. They will be discussed with the intention of showing that this approach could lead to a synthesis of many systems of treatment which have hitherto been widely regarded as being mutually exclusive (Chapter 4).

ASSOCIATED HANDICAPS

Brain damage in cerebral palsy may also be responsible for special sense defects of vision and hearing, abnormalities of speech and language and aberrations of perception. Perceptual defects or *agnosias* are difficulties in recognising objects or symbols, even though sensation as such is not impaired, and the patient can prove by other means to know or have known what the object or symbol is. There may also be *apraxias*, some of which are also called visuomotor defects. This means that the child is unable to perform certain movements even though there is no paralysis, because the patterns or 'engrams' have been lost or have not developed. Apraxia can involve movements of the limbs, face, eyes, tongue or be specifically restricted to such acts as writing, drawing, and construction or even dressing. In other words there seems to be a problem in 'motor planning' in those children who are apraxic. Cerebral palsied children may also have various behaviour problems such as distractibility and hyperkinesis which are based on the organic brain damage. All these defects result in various learning problems and difficulties in communication. In addition there may also be mental defect or epilepsy.

Not every child has some or all of these associated handicaps. Even if the handicap were only physical, the resulting paucity of movement would prevent the child from fully exploring the environment. He is therefore limited in the acquisition of sensations and perceptions of everyday things. A child may then *appear* to have defects of perception, but these may not be organic but caused by lack of experience. The same lack of everyday experiences retards the development of language and affects the child's speech. His general understanding may suffer so that he appears to be mentally retarded. This can go so far that normal intelligence has been camouflaged by severe physical handicap. Furthermore the lack of movement can affect the general behaviour of the child. Thus some abnormal behaviour may be due to the lack of satisfying emotional and social experiences for which movement is necessary. It is therefore important for any therapist to recognise that motor function cannot be isolated from other functions and that she is treating a child who is not solely physically but multiply handicapped.

AETIOLOGY

There are many causes of the brain damage, including abnormal development of the brain, anoxia, intracranial bleeding, excessive neonatal jaundice, trauma and infection. These have been extensively discussed in the medical literature [1–12]. The therapist is, however, rarely guided by the aetiology in her treatment planning. In some cases the cause is not certain and in many cases knowing the cause does not necessarily indicate a specific diagnosis or specific treatment. Nevertheless, the therapist should acquaint herself with the history of the case. Many of these children have been affected from infancy and have been difficult to feed and handle. This may easily have influenced the parent–child relationships. Furthermore the history may sometimes give an indication of the prognosis, e.g. with marked microcephaly the prognosis would be poor.

CLINICAL PICTURE AND DEVELOPMENT

It is important to recognise that the causes of cerebral palsy take place in the prenatal, perinatal, and postnatal periods. In all cases, it is an immature nervous system which suffers the insult and the nervous system afterwards continues to develop in the presence of the damage. The therapist must therefore not think of herself as treating an upper motor neurone lesion in a 'little adult' nor can she regard the problem solely as one of retardation in development. What the therapist faces is a complex situation of pathological symptoms within the context of a developing child [13–43]. There are three main aspects to the clinical picture:
1 Retardation in the development of new skills expected at the child's chronological age.
2 Persistence of infantile behaviour in all functions, including infantile reflex reactions.
3 Performance of various functions in patterns never seen in normal babies and children. This is because the pathological symptoms of upper motor neurone lesions such as hypertonus, hypotonus, involuntary movements and pathological reflexes are present.

In order to recognise abnormal motor and general behaviour, the therapist should know what a normal child does and how he does it at the various stages of his development [20, 21, 22, 23]. Information on each handicapped child's developmental levels should be sought from the consultants and other members of the cerebral palsy team. Reference will have to be made to the extensive literature on the field of child development.

Although normal child development is the basis on which the abnormal development is appreciated, it does not follow that assessment and treatment should rely upon a strict adherence to normal developmental schedules. Even 'normal' children show many variations from the 'normal' developmental sequences and patterns of development which have been derived from the *average* child. The cerebral palsied child will show additional variations due to neurological and mechanical difficulties. If one considers, say, the normal developmental scales of gross motor development, the cerebral palsied child has frequently achieved abilities at one level of development, omitted abilities at another level and only partially achieved motor abilities at still other levels. There is thus a scatter of abilities.

If the gross motor development is generally considered to be around a given age, the development of hand function, speech and language, social and emotional and intellectual levels may all be at different ages. None of these ages may necessarily coincide with the child's chronological age.

Therefore the developmental schedules in normal child development should only be used as *guidelines* in treatment and adaptation should be made for each child's handicaps and individuality (Chapter 4).

More attention is usually given to motor development rather than other avenues of development, as it is the motor handicap which characterises cerebral palsy. Here again, the therapist should remember that abnormal motor behaviour may interfere with other functions. Each area of development—such as gross motor, manipulation, speech and language, perception, social and emotional and mental—interacts as well as each having its own pattern or avenue of development. Therefore a total habilitation programme is necessary and should be planned to deal with the total development of the child.

Whilst aiming at the maximum function possible, the therapists concerned must take account of the *damaged* nervous system and adjust their expectations of achievements by the child which involves:

1 Late acquisition of motor skills and slow rate of progress from one stage to the next.
2 A smaller variety of skills than in the normal child.
3 Variations in normal sequences of skills.
4 Abnormal patterns of the skills.

Furthermore, the potential for function is dependent not only on the defects present, but also on the emotional and social adjustment of the child, his personality and 'drive' as well as his intelligence.

CHANGE IN CLINICAL PICTURE

As the lesion is in a developing nervous system the clinical picture is clearly not a static set of signs and symptoms for treatment. But whilst the lesion itself is non-progressive its manifestations change as the nervous system matures. As more is demanded of the nervous system the degree of the handicap appears to be greater. For example, a 3-year-old is expected to do more than a baby, and therefore his failures are greater for the same lesion.

In addition, the pathological symptoms may develop with the years. Spasticity may increase, involuntary movements may only appear at the age of 2 or 3 years, and ataxia may only be diagnosed when the child walks or when grasp is expected to become more accurate. Diagnoses may change as the baby develops to childhood, and especially as the child becomes more active. Later, especially in adolescence, growth and increase in weight contribute to apparent deterioration as the child matures.

Treatment minimises the aggravation of symptoms. The earlier treatment is started the more opportunity is given for whatever potential there may be for developing any normal abilities and for decreasing the defects.

Although the clinical picture is known to change with the years it is not yet possible to predict the natural history of the condition in each particular child. Infants and babies with marked early neurological signs may later prove to be only mildly affected, or even normal. On the other hand, apparently mildly affected ones may become progressively worse with the years. It is therefore difficult to prove the value of every early treatment. Nevertheless until we know which babies are going to 'come right' on their own, it is better to let them have the benefit of treatment so that any potentials for improvement are not lost. Despite the controversy as to the value of early treatment, there is moreover no doubt about its importance to the parents, who receive a great deal of practical advice and support from the therapists. Whilst medical practitioners are watching the development of the child in order to make a reliable diagnosis, the parents have to live with that child throughout each day of those months and years.

CLASSIFICATION

Numerous classifications and subclassifications have been proposed by different authorities [1–12], but none of these diagnostic labels suffice to formulate adequate treatment plans. The therapist must also have a detailed assessment based primarily on motor functions, in order to work out a treatment programme.

There are classifications of topography and types of cerebral palsy.

The topographical classifications frequently used are as follows:

Quadriplegia: Involvement of four limbs. Double hemiplegia is also used meaning that the arms are more affected than the legs and that there may be a congenital suprabulbar palsy.

Diplegia: Involvement of four limbs with the legs more affected than the arms.

Paraplegia: Involvement of both legs.

Triplegia: Involvement of three limbs.

Hemiplegia: One side of the body is affected.

Monoplegia: One limb is affected.

These topographical classifications are imprecise in that the other limbs may be slightly involved as well. The therapist should always consider whether or not she needs to include the 'uninvolved' limbs in her treatment.

The hands of a paraplegic, for example, may need training in finer coordination or perhaps the other side of a hemiplegic may require treatment. The quadriplegics are often asymmetrical, with some of the limbs more obviously affected than the others. Triplegias and hemiplegias may really be quadriplegias. A pure monoplegia is almost non-existent.

The types of involvement are spasticity, rigidity, athetosis or hypotonicity. This latter called 'atonic' cerebral palsy rarely remains hypotonic. These floppy babies usually become spastic, athetoid or ataxic. Athetoids and ataxics are mostly quadriplegic, but there is occasionally a hemiathetoid.

The classifications into types of cerebral palsy vary in different clinics but generally the main types are the *spastic*, the *athetoid* and the *ataxic*. Once again these classifications are not clear cut and the therapist may have to treat symptoms of one type of cerebral palsy in another type. The predominant symptoms will contribute to the diagnostic type referred for treatment.

THE SPASTIC

Main motor characteristics are:

Hypertonus of the 'clasp-knife' variety. If the spastic muscles are stretched at a particular speed they respond in an exaggerated fashion. They contract, blocking the movement. This hyperactive stretch reflex may occur at the beginning, middle or near the end of the range of movement. There are increased tendon jerks, occasional clonus and other signs of upper motor neurone lesions.

Abnormal postures These are usually associated with the antigravity muscles which are extensors in the leg and the flexors in the arm. The therapist will find *many* variations on this especially when the child reaches different levels of development [14]. Common abnormal postures in supine, prone, sitting, standing, walking and in hand function are described in Chapters 6 and 8.

The abnormal postures are held by tight spastic muscle groups whose antagonists are weak, or apparently weak in that they cannot overcome the tight pull of the spastic muscles and so correct the abnormal postures. There are various other causes of abnormal postures which are discussed in Chapter 8. Abnormal postures appear as unfixed deformities which may become fixed deformities or contractures.

Changes in hypertonus and postures may occur with excitement, fear or anxiety which increases muscle tension. Shifts in hypertonus occur in the same affected parts of the body or from one part of the body to another in, say, stimulation of abnormal reactions such as 'associated reactions' or remnants of tonic reflex activity. Changes in hypertonus are seen with changes of position in some children. Position of the head and neck may affect the distribution of hypertonus. The latter are due to abnormal reflexes which may sometimes be found in these children. Sudden movements, rather than slow movements, increase hypertonus.

Hypertonus may be either spasticity or rigidity. The overlap between the two is almost impossible to differentiate. Rigidity is recognised by a 'plastic' or continuous resistance to passive stretch throughout the full range of motion. This 'lead pipe' rigidity differs from spasticity as spasticity offers resistance at a point or small part of the passive range of motion. For treatment planning the type of hypertonus is rarely important and techniques for motor development and prevention of deformity are the same.

Voluntary movement Spasticity does not mean paralysis. Voluntary motion is present and may be laboured. There may be weakness in the initiation of motion or during movement at different parts of its range. If spasticity is decreased or removed by treatment or drugs, the spastic muscles may be found to be strong, or may be weak. Once spasticity is decreased the antagonists may also be stronger once they no longer have to overcome the resistance of tight spastic muscles. However, in time these antagonists may have become weak with disuse.

The groups of muscles or 'chains' of muscles used in the movement patterns are different from those used in normal children of the same age. Either the muscles which work in association with each other are stereotyped and are occasionally seen in the normal child, usually at an infantile level of movement, or the association of muscles is abnormal. For example, hip extension-adduction-internal rotation is used in creeping movements or in the push-off in walking but many other combinations must be used during the full execution of creeping and walking. This may be impossible in spastics who continue to use the same pattern at all times in the motor skill. Another example is shoulder flexion-adduction with some external rotation for feeding or combing one's hair in the normal arm pattern. In the case of the spastic, the arm pattern is usually flexion-adduction with *internal* rotation and *pronation* of the elbow. In taking a step in walking the normal pattern is flexion-adduction-external rotation at the hip, whereas the spastic pattern is frequently flexion-adduction-*internal* rotation of the hip. Other abnormal movement patterns occur as co-contraction of the agonist with the antagonist, instead of the normal relaxation of the antagonist. This blocks movement or makes it laboured. There are usually mass movements in that the child is unable to move an isolated joint. This absence of discrete movement is a characteristic feature of many spastics. Clearly there is not the smooth, coordinated, effortless and subconscious action of muscle patterns seen in normal motor skills.

General
1 Intelligence varies, tending to be lower than in athetoids.

2 Perceptual problems especially of spatial relationships are more common in spastics than in athetoids.
3 Sensory loss occasionally occurs in the spastic hemiplegic hand and visual field. Growth of the hemiplegic limbs is less than in the unaffected side.
4 Epilepsy is more common than in athetoids.

THE ATHETOID

Main motor characteristics are:

Involuntary movements—athetosis. These are bizarre, purposeless movements which may be uncontrollable. The involuntary movements may be slow or fast; they may be writhing, jerky, tremor, swiping or rotary patterns or they may be unpatterned. They are present at rest in some children. The involuntary motion is increased by excitement, any form of insecurity, and the effort to make a voluntary movement or even to tackle a mental problem. Factors which decrease athetosis are fatigue, drowsiness, fever, prone lying or the child's attention being deeply held. Athetosis may be present in all parts of the body including the face and tongue. Athetosis may only appear in hands or feet or in proximal joints or in both distal and proximal joints.

Voluntary movements   These are possible but there may be an initial delay before the movement is begun. The involuntary movement may partially or totally disrupt the willed movement making it uncoordinated. There is a lack of finer movements and weakness.

Hypertonia or hypotonia   Either may exist or there may be fluctuations of tone. Athetoids are sometimes called 'tension and non-tension' types. There may be dystonia or twisting of the head, trunk or limbs. Sudden spasms of flexion or extension could occur. The hypertonia is a rigidity but occasionally spasticity may be present in the athetoid quadriplegias. Fluctuating tone sometimes occurs with fluctuations of mood or emotions.

The Athetoid dance   Some athetoids are unable to maintain weight on their feet and continually withdraw their feet upwards or upwards and outwards in an athetoid dance. They may take weight on one foot whilst pawing or scraping the ground in a withdrawal motion with the other leg. This has been attributed to a conflict between grasp and withdrawal reflexes. This conflict of reflexes may also be seen in the hands [5, 37, 38].

Paralysis of gaze movements may occur so that athetoids may find it difficult to look upwards and sometimes also to close their eyes voluntarily.

Athetoids change with time They may be floppy in babyhood and only exhibit the involuntary movements when they reach 2 or 3 years of age. Adult athetoids do not appear hypotonic but have muscle tension. Muscle tension also seems to be increased in an effort to control involuntary movements.

Subclassifications of athetoids vary from clinic to clinic. It is therefore particularly inaccurate to discuss the 'treatment of athetoids'. As mentioned above any classification changes with time. The therapist should treat the symptoms found rather than the subclassification.

General
1 Intelligence is frequently good and may be very high. Mental defect also occurs.
2 Hearing loss of a specific high frequency type is associated with athetoids caused by kernicterus.
3 'Drive' and outgoing personalities are often observed among athetoids. Emotional lability is more frequent than in other cerebral palsies.

THE ATAXIC

Main motor characteristics are:

Disturbances of balance There is poor fixation of the head, trunk, shoulder and pelvic girdles. Some ataxics overcompensate for this instability by having excessive balance-saving reactions in the arms. Instability is also found in athetoids and spastics (see below).

Voluntary movements are present but clumsy or uncoordinated. The child overreaches or underreaches for an object and is said to have 'dysmetria'. This inaccurate limb movement in relation to its objective may also be accompanied by intention tremor. Poor fine hand movements occur.

Hypotonia is usual. Ataxia may be present in the hypertonic cases as well.

Nystagmus may exist.

General
1 Intelligence is often low. Visual, hearing, perception problems may occur.
2 Mentally subnormal, 'clumsy' intelligent children may present as ataxics as well as a mixed group of cerebral palsied children who may show any of the multiple handicaps already mentioned. A 'pure' ataxic is rare.

COMMON FEATURES IN ALL TYPES OF CEREBRAL PALSY

The classification into types of cerebral palsy tends to obscure the fact that there are important motor features which are common to all types. For instance, all cerebral palsied children are retarded in motor development. However the symptoms of the different types of cerebral palsy, such as hypertonus and the various involuntary movements only play a part in this disturbance of development. Retarded or abnormal development of the postural-balance mechanisms or postural reflexes disturbs the motor development. Another common feature is the presence of certain abnormal reflexes which have no predilection for a specific type of cerebral palsy.

POSTURAL MECHANISMS (POSTURAL REFLEXES)

The inability to maintain posture and balance is most obvious in the athetoids and the ataxics, but is as much a cause of the physical handicap in the spastic type. Even if the spasticity were removed, the child would still be physically handicapped (page 39). The postural reflexes or postural mechanisms are neurological mechanisms which help to maintain posture and equilibrium and which are involved in locomotion. They have been described by various neurological workers. Purdon Martin [29, 30] has drawn on their work and, together with his own observations, presents a clear functional scheme which is described in Chapter 4 and related to development training and deformity in Chapters 5, 6 and 8.

The postural reactions are an intrinsic part of motor skills. When they are absent or abnormal they lead to absent or abnormal motor skills. As the child acquires the different motor skills at various levels of development, he is in fact developing these postural mechanisms. Paediatric neurologists have studied the approximate ages at which these neurological mechanisms appear [13–16, 31–41]. They are sometimes called 'automatisms' which appear with maturation. Milani has grouped them into *righting reactions*, *parachute reactions* and *tilt reactions* which appear at different developmental levels. Others have grouped them differently. Irrespective of the terminology used, the therapist should know what these reactions are and in what general sequence they are expected in development so that she can stimulate them in the treatment and management of the child. The postural mechanisms cannot be isolated from voluntary movements. Unfortunately some clinicians have overemphasised and isolated the problems of voluntary movement in the cerebral palsied child. The weakness and other abnormalities of voluntary movement have already been mentioned under the types of cerebral palsy. It is, however, important to understand that weakness of voluntary movement can also be bound up with the inadequacy of the postural mechanisms. When a child makes a voluntary movement, he has to maintain his balance as he does so. If equilibrium is inadequate the child may not be able to initiate a movement, or if he manages to carry out the movement on a background of unstable posture, that movement tends to be clumsy or uncoordinated. It is interesting to observe that during the development of hand function there is a period when the baby's hand skills are imprecise because his sitting balance has not been reliably established. It is therefore pointless for the therapist to train movements of arms or legs if the head and trunk are not being stabilised, with special methods.

One kind of weakness found in all cerebral palsied children is either of the muscles of head, trunk, shoulder and pelvic girdle or all of them. These are the muscles which are activated by the postural mechanisms. If these mechanisms are absent and the muscles cannot be activated, it is hardly surprising that they should be weak. One of the many reasons for floppy babies could be a lack of stimulation of the postural mechanisms. In cerebral palsied children floppiness of the head and trunk are also seen together with hypertonic limbs. This lack of development of head and trunk control is usually attributed to retardation of motor development. But this is in effect due to retarded development of the mechanisms of postural fixation of the head and trunk.

ABNORMAL REFLEXES (see Table 5.2. page 56)

Besides the desirable postural reactions, there are also reflexes which are undesirable. Many such pathological reflexes have been described in cerebral palsied children of all types. Diagnostic reflexes such as the tendon jerks, however, are of little relevance to treatment planning. Those reflexes which concern the therapist are some of the infantile or primitive reflexes. These are reflexes which are present in the normal newborn and which become integrated or disappear as the baby matures. In cerebral palsied children infantile reflexes are still present long after the ages when they should have become integrated within the nervous system. Whilst there are many infantile reflexes, those of most interest to the therapist are the Moro reflex, the palmar and plantar grasp reflexes, automatic stepping, excessive neck righting reflex, positive supporting and feeding reflexes.

There are also the tonic reflexes, which are the tonic labyrinthine reflexes (TLR), the asymmetrical tonic neck reflex (ATNR) and the symmetrical tonic neck reflexes (STNR). Some neurologists group these tonic reflexes amongst the infantile reflexes whereas other argue that they are not present in the normal infant and are always pathological. These tonic reflexes are sometimes called 'postural reflexes' but they are *abnormal* postural reflexes and should not be confused with the normal postural mechanisms [44–46].

The principle of treatment which therapists should follow in relation to the complicated collection of reflexes is *not* to go 'reflex hunting'. Reflexes only concern the therapist when they interfere with motor function and speech. This does *not* always occur. The approach is to examine the function of the child first and only when abnormality has been detected, to then consider whether *one* of the reasons for this abnormality seems to be a pathological or primitive reflex.

MOTOR DELAY

Cerebral palsy consists of both motor delay and motor disorder. There are many other conditions which present similar problems of motor delay or of delay and disorder. All these conditions are also called the *Developmental Disabilities* [43].

They may be due to:

Mental subnormality which is caused by various metabolic disorders, chromosome anomalies, leucodystrophies, microcephaly and other abnormalities of the skull and brain, endocrine disorders and the causes of brain damage given for the cerebral palsies.

Deprivation of normal stimulation associated with social, economic and emotional problems.

Malnutrition alone, but usually together with deprived environments. Once malnutrition is treated, lack of normal stimulation may still retard the child's development.

The presence of non-motor handicaps which may lead to motor delay, e.g. blindness, severe perceptual defects, apraxias, as well as mental handicap mentioned above. Children with delay in any developmental area may have an associated delay in motor development.

Presence of motor handicaps other than the cerebral palsies For example spina bifida, the myopathies, myelopathies and various progressive neurological diseases and congenital deformities may obviously delay development, e.g. hand function has been delayed in children with spina bifida [25].

Principles of treatment, and organisation of treatment will be similar to that discussed in this and the next chapter. Although differences will be obvious in the discussions of the spastic, the athetoid and the ataxic, these problems may also be found in the mentally subnormal and other neurological conditions. *Specific problems* in the conditions above are considered in other publications.

SUMMARY

Whilst it is difficult to summarise the principles of treatment concisely, the following points may be useful provided they are studied after reading chapters 1 and 4.

1 The child should be seen as being not only physically but multiply handicapped. In addition to motor dysfunction, associated handicaps may occur because of either brain damage, or lack of experiences due to inadequate movement, or both aspects combined.

2 Treatment should be aimed at the neurological mechanisms of posture, balance and movement, supplemented by procedures for muscles and joints when necessary.

3 There should not be a rigid adherence to particular diagnostic classifications in treatment programmes, and aetiology may not influence the treatment in cerebral palsy.

4 Emphasis should be given to training various postural mechanisms which are absent or abnormal in all types of cerebral palsy, or absent in any developmental motor delay.

5 Treatment should also provide for features of the motor disorder such as hypertonicity, hypotonicity, involuntary movements, weakness, abnormal patterns of voluntary movements and abnormal reflexes.

6 The therapist should deal with abnormal reflexes only in those cases where they directly disrupt function.

7 The therapist must deal with a complex situation of pathological symptoms within the context of a *developing* child in the cerebral palsies and other motor disorders.

8 Developmental schedules of normal child development should only be used as guidelines and adaptations made to each child.

9 Treatment should commence as early as possible.

10 Treatment plans should be reviewed periodically to take account of changes in the clinical picture as the child grows older.

CHAPTER 2

ORGANISATION OF TREATMENT

In translating the fundamental principles of treatment into practice special attention should be paid to the following aspects [1–18].

TREATMENT PLANNING

Treatment must be carefully planned as follows:
1   A total assessment of the child must be obtained.
2   A specific examination for the particular therapy, i.e. physiotherapy, occupational therapy or speech therapy, should be made.
3   Aims of treatment are worked out on the basis of the above.
4   Techniques of treatment are selected according to the problems of the individual child.
5   Periodic reassessments of the child's progress is required.

The time required to assess each child varies. *Full* assessment is not always possible on the first meeting. Firstly, if he is not accustomed to the new environment or is distressed in any way he may not reveal his true potential. Secondly, if he is given some treatment he may then reveal an underlying potential.

Besides the consideration of the child's abilities and disabilities, each therapist should also observe the individual personality of the child and his family. Although the social worker and psychologist concentrate on these aspects, it is important to have observations on the emotional and social aspects from all who are making relationships with the child and his family. Naturally the therapist is involved in these relationships.

The aims of treatment are worked out based on the assessment. In general the aims of treatment will centre on:
1   Developing forms of communication (speech, gesture, writing or sign language, typing).
2   Developing independence in the daily activities of feeding, dressing, washing and toiletting.
3   Developing some form of locomotion.

The selection of techniques is also based on the total and specific assessments. Observation of the child is important in order to see whether there is any response to the methods chosen, which can then be continued, modified or discarded. Techniques are selected from any system of treatment according to the child. This eclectic approach is elaborated in the chapters that follow.

Periodic reassessment of the child's progress and thus the value of the total and specific programmes, is essential [20–22].

Records should be kept of the assessments, treatment and progress.

TEAMWORK

The total assessment and treatment or habilitation programme for each child will depend on a team of specialists. The ideal team consists of medical consultants in paediatrics, neurology, psychiatry, orthopaedics, oto-laryngology and ophthalmology with physiotherapists, occupational therapists, speech therapists, teachers, social workers, psychologists, and the parents. Excellent progress has nevertheless been made by patients when cared for by a much smaller and well integrated team as long as all aspects of the child are considered. It is preferable to limit the numbers of adults assessing and treating the young child. Whenever referral must be made to a consultant, it is helpful to the child if he can be seen in a familiar environment such as his home or cerebral palsy unit, and also he should be with someone he knows and likes. In the day-to-day therapy, the child is usually more responsive to the same few adults. Babies are best handled by one therapist with any special additional advice given to her and the parents by the other specialists.

Effective teamwork does not consist of separate assessments and special-ised training of specific handicaps by each team member and then adding up the list of handicaps as if they equal a 'whole child'. Although specialised work is important, attention must also be given to any interaction of dif-ferent defects. In addition assets in one function may be used to develop another different and inadequate function. For example, speech may rein-force movement, motor activities may stimulate speech, movement may be used to train perception, perceptual activities and motion may develop language and so on. It is therefore unsound for any therapist to isolate her-self in her own specific area.

Thus, physiotherapists, speech therapists, occupational therapists and teachers must not only concentrate on the aspects of the child's behaviour relevant to their professions, all must explore how their speciality *overlaps* with the others. This is carried out by an interchange of information and where necessary by showing each other possible ways of handling each child. These practical recommendations must also be shown to the parents, residental care staff, voluntary helpers and nursing staff. When laymen and new staff are being instructed the explanations should be simple and technical language should be avoided.

All those caring for the child should learn the following:
1 Which postures and movements including patterns of locomotion to encourage so that they become more reliable with practice and the child becomes less handicapped.

2 What undesirable motor behaviour to discourage. This will also prevent deformities which block further development.

3 Which positions make it easier for the child to move and communicate.

4 How to communicate with the child.

5 How to develop language and stimulate speech.

6 Which sensory and perceptual experiences to encourage.

7 Which pieces of equipment to use to facilitate function, what furniture and which aids are indicated for feeding, dressing, washing and toiletting; when to dispense with aids.

8 How to carry the child if necessary.

9 Which toys and play activities to use in order to motivate the above.

All these aspects of specialised information are individual and interwoven. Good total handling of the child by those who care for him reinforces any specific training in all situations and prevents isolation of the child's different areas of function. Treatment (pp. 69–206) will therefore include not only physiotherapy methods for the primary motor handicap but also practical recommendations to other members of the cerebral palsy team.

The interdisciplinary treatment of physiotherapist, occupational therapists, speech therapists, teachers and social workers is facilitated by:

1 Staff conferences.

2 Informal discussions over tea and elsewhere.

3 Visits to one another's rooms for observation and treatment of each person's own patients.

4 Combined treatments by different therapists or working with the teachers in the classroom or playground, with the social workers, health visitors on home visits, or with nurses in hospital wards.

5 Interdisciplinary group activities or therapeutic group work. (See Chapter 9.)

CONTINUOUS MANAGEMENT

Treatment cannot be seen as only a half-hour or so session a day or three times a week. The nervous system is responsive to what is happening all the time and not just during short intensive stimulation called 'therapy'. For example the important stimulations of the postural reflexes are carried out by specific techniques in a treatment session. If the child is then fully supported for the rest of the day there is no activation of any postural reflexes and it is difficult for them to become established and lead to the child, say, sitting or standing on his own. If deformities are being counteracted in a treatment session they should then not be accentuated by abnormal positions for the rest of the day and night.

It is therefore important to recognise that correct handling and suitable equipment throughout the day is 'treatment' as well as what is done during specialised therapy sessions. Many children have made improvement with good continuous management even without specific treatment sessions.

In many cases, it is controversial whether greater improvement will be obtained if treatment sessions are also included. I believe in including treatment sessions whenever possible. The sessions may have to be omitted or decreased where there is a severe shortage of trained therapists or when there are difficulties in having regular attendance of the child at a Treatment Centre.

The therapist must thus allocate her time to treating the child and to teaching others to handle the child in the best possible way.

The ideas on the correct management of the child listed above should be given to parents and others as soon as possible. The therapist may also have to teach specific treatment techniques or exercises for the baby or child, to those parents who can manage it.

SENSORY-MOTOR EXPERIENCES

The value of early management and treatment of handicapped babies is that the resulting general stimulation of various functions decreases the inevitable lack of everyday experiences of normal child development. The sooner the baby can be helped to move, the sooner he can explore, the sooner he can be helped to communicate, and the sooner he can therefore acquire information. The therapist is in fact contributing to the education of the child in the broadest sense.

Whenever motor function is being increased this motor function must also be used to acquire sensations of ordinary objects in the home. The child must be encouraged to feel textures, shapes, temperatures and other sensations. He should be helped to move through space, to go 'under, over, inside and outside' so that he both experiences this and learns the words for it. Visit to shops, the zoo, the country and other places are an important part of his therapy as well as his education, provided that advantage is taken of these situations for motivating movement and speech. During these visits time and patience should be given to let him use the movements and the speech that he has acquired.

Various play activities with sand, water and many materials of different shapes and textures not only motivate movements, but the movements used in playing help him acquire sensory and perceptual experiences. These basic sensory motor activities are basic learning experiences and thus therapy and education become integrated.

OBTAINING COOPERATION OF BABIES AND CHILDREN

Time is often needed for the child to accept the new environment, the treatment situation, and crucially, a new person, the therapist.

At first it is valuable to have the mother present to reassure the child—

and the mother. If she has to learn how to handle and treat the child or baby, she should always be present with the therapist. It is, however, also necessary to wean the child from the mother's presence, especially if the child is overprotected or being prepared for nursery school. When his mother is out of the treatment room he should be shown where she is waiting for him. He might also keep one of her possessions in the room to reassure him. At this stage and later, one-way windows are recommended in order to let mothers continue to observe treatment.

The child may also accept the therapist more readily if the parents are seen to do so. At the first meeting the therapist might spend most of the time talking with them, whilst leaving the child to play nearby. She could watch the child unobtrusively. When the therapist herself plays with the child she will not only make friends with him but skilfully use the play to obtain information on his behaviour. Well chosen toys, action songs, and any motivation of movements or speech are important in helping the child to adjust to being treated, as well as contributing to assessment and treatment.

If the child is new to a Centre, the therapist should give him time to settle down in his new playroom or classroom. She could play with him in the classroom or the playground and once rapport is obtained invite him into her own room. In some cases it helps the child if at first he is allowed to watch his new therapist treating other children.

Babies and young children may cry when first treated. They do not necessarily want to make independent movements and find it easier to be 'coddled'. The methods that relax hypertonus give them odd, unaccustomed experiences and they may not welcome the stranger 'interfering' with them. As early treatment is important and as babies almost always learn to accept the necessary handling in time, the therapist should not stop treatment. She can initially limit its length, use more play and songs, ask the mother to practice more of her handling. If possible treatment in the baby's own home is desirable for those babies who find the strangeness of the clinic, the therapist and the treatment too much to tolerate. However if, toddlers can have treatment at a Centre just before entering its nursery school it may help them in their initial adjustment to the Centre.

Treating the baby and the young child does not require formal cooperation from the child and under the age of 3 years this should not be expected. Through handling the child with the use of sensory stimuli, through the use of toys and equipment the child is stimulated to move without any verbal instruction. Words are used but more to develop language than to elicit any motor response at this stage.

The older child who will not cooperate may be showing a self-assertiveness and rebellion to adults which may be a normal part of his emotional development. Such children often respond better if treated with one or two others about their age or in a larger group. A change or interruption of treatment may be needed for a period whilst some new incentive is sought. Games, swimming, dancing and other activities in physical education should be discussed with the physical training instructor and the corrective procedures for the older child incorporated in them. If any child is particularly uncooperative, it is important to analyse the reason for this with all members of the cerebral palsy team.

Obtaining the cooperation of the child is also helped by planning and carrying out the treatment to incorporate newer understanding of learning processes developed by psychologists and teachers.

LEARNING PROCESSES

Speech therapy and occupational therapy obviously overlap with education in drawing on learning techniques. Physiotherapy has 'grown-up' predominently within the fields of neurophysiology and orthopaedics. Physiotherapy involves specialised neurophysiological stimulation of the mechanisms of posture, balance and movement. But it is not by neurophysiology alone that one treats these children. Physiotherapists also should draw on the fields of psychology and education.

Some examples of learning techniques which are commonly used are the following:

Repetition is required for learning and therefore activities in therapy should be repeated during the treatment sessions and selected activities in the all-day management of the child.

Motivation of the child should be attempted through the use of play, toys, interesting equipment, music, various social situations and through well-designed clinics, schools and playgrounds. Some social situations which motivate many children are group treatments, group games and free play group as well as a good family.

There are children, especially the older and/or the intelligent child who motivate themselves to work hard in and out of treatment. These children will have less need than others of external motivation aids or the use of play, toys, etc. in order to achieve skills.

Further incentives for learning are to provide 'rewards' for those children who have the capacity to 'work hard'. This does not only mean rewarding him with a sweet after he has tried hard in treatment. In fact this should not always be used. The achievement of a task a little beyond the child's apparent ability is reward in itself. Treatment should be so graded that this can occur. The child is also rewarded by the approval of his peers, his parents and his therapist. Other incentives are keeping a progress chart, collecting 'stars' for achievements or receiving other presentations. It may also help to have competition with similarly handicapped children.

Incentives should be devised so as to be meaningful to the child, taking account of his intelligence and particular background.

However systems of rewards, direct or indirect, may alone not prove effective with all children. In some cases the therapist will have to supervise the child closely and subtly exert pressure to obtain, as far as possible, 'hard work'.

Cues for learning should be clear in treatment. These cues are given by the therapist with her hands as she uses sensory (afferent) stimuli for motor responses: in her verbal instructions and when asking a child to imitate what she does or what another child does in the room or in a group treatment.

Instructions should be given according to the child's level of comprehension, which depends not only on his intellectual level but also on his social class. Sentence structure should be simple and short for young and for mentally retarded children. Verbal instructions should be precise. In physiotherapy it is advisable to use an operative word for movement such as 'bend, bend, bend' or 'push, push, push'. In this way the child also learns the meaning of the word through the action that goes with it.

When training a motor skill it is helpful to accompany the movement with speech. Thus when training a child to stand up from a chair, the child and the therapist, or the therapist alone might verbalise the skill involved by saying: 'Put your feet flat, go forward over your feet and stand up.' The value of this technique can be appreciated when one remembers that even normal people often verbalise their movements when they are learning a new skill such as playing tennis, driving a car, ice skating or piano playing. Thus in learning a tennis stroke one initially says to oneself: 'Arm up, back and through'. Once the skill is learnt and becomes automatic, the verbalisation is no longer needed.

In order that the cues for learning are clear, account must obviously be taken of any non-motor or associated handicaps in the child. Members of the treatment-education team should obviously advise each other. The therapist should know that if the child is deaf, she should talk to him with her face in a good light, at his eye level. If he has visual problems she should emphasise the sensory stimuli usually used in therapy techniques, use verbal reinforcement and other learning cues for sensory-motor understanding. If the child has perceptual or praxic problems the verbalisation should be particularly clear, concentrating on the sensory, motor and perceptual areas which are not affected. If the child is mentally defective, the range of activities should be decreased, simplified and frequently repeated. Should the child not understand spoken words whilst being otherwise intelligent as in a 'receptive aphasia' then the therapist should use sensory, perceptual and motor activities in addition to speech. All team members should use the same words to label activities, so that there is consistency.

Active treatment is important [24, 86] as the child learns best what he does himself. Some passive correction in physiotherapy and during the day and night management is inevitably needed for deformities, but these should also be actively corrected.

A sense of achievement spurs the child on to the next stage of development. Therefore treatment should not comprise a series of difficult tasks intended to overcome his defects, but at which he always fails. Activities must be planned and graded so that he does experience success. This experience reinforces progress [24].

The home environment should be conducive to the child's learning and development. The practical advice and good relationships with parents will support them and improve the atmosphere in the home.

Behaviour modification experts should be consulted.

CHAPTER 3

OUTLINE OF TREATMENT APPROACHES

There are many systems of treatment for cerebral palsy [25, 67–73]. Although these therapeutic approaches were devised for the cerebral palsies, many of them are also used for treatment of children with other conditions of developmental delay and for adults with neurological defects. It is not the purpose of this chapter to describe each system in full detail and reference should be made to the literature and study observations of each system in practice. The author presents the essence of each system after many personal observations, discussions, practical work and reading of the work of the originators.

MUSCLE EDUCATION AND BRACES

W. M. Phelps [26–28] an orthopaedic surgeon in Baltimore, was one of the pioneers in the treatment of cerebral palsy who encouraged physiotherapists, occupational therapists and speech therapists to form themselves into cerebral palsy habilitation teams. The main points in his treatment approach were:

Specific diagnostic classification of each child as a basis for specific treatment methods. He diagnosed five types of cerebral palsy and many subclassifications.

Fifteen modalities were described and specific combinations of these modalities were used for the specific type of cerebral palsy.
The modalities (methods) were:
1 Massage for hypotonic muscles, but contraindicated in spastics and athetoids.
2 Passive motion through joint range for mobilising joints and demonstrating to the child the movement required. Speed of movement is slower for spastics, increased for rigidity.
3 Active assisted motion.
4 Active motion.
5 Resisted motion followed according to the child's capability.
The above modalities were used for obtaining modalities 6, 8, 10 and 12.
6 Conditioned motion is recommended for babies, young children and mentally retarded children.

7 Confused motion or synergistic motion which involves resistance to a muscle group in order to contract an inactive muscle group in the same synergy. Mass movements such as the extensor thrust or the flexion withdrawal reflex are usually used. For example, using the hip-knee flexion dorsiflexion synergy, inactive dorsiflexors are stimulated by resistance given to hip flexors. Confused motion is further discussed in the sections on deformity.

8 Combined motion is training motion of more than one joint, such as a shoulder and elbow flexion using modalities 2, 3, 4, 5.

9 Relaxation techniques used are those of Fink's conscious 'letting go' of the body and its parts [71], and Jacobson's method of tensing and relaxing parts of the body [29]. These methods are mainly used with athetoids. They attempt to lie still or relaxed or use contract-relax relaxation for grimacing and other involuntary motion.

10 Movement from relaxation is conscious control of movements once relaxation has been achieved. It is mainly used for children to control involuntary movements.

11 Rest. Periods of rest are suggested for athetoids and spastics.

12 Reciprocation is training movement of one leg after the other in a bicycling pattern in lying, crawling, knee walking, and stepping.

13 Balance. Training of sitting balance and standing in braces.

14 Reach and grasp and release used for training of hand function.

15 Skills of daily living such as feeding, dressing, washing and toiletting. Many aids were devised by the occupational therapists.

Braces or calipers These appliances were designed and developed by Phelps. He prescribed special braces to correct deformity, to obtain the upright position and to control athetosis. The bracing is extensive and worn for many years. The children are taught to stand and step in long leg braces with pelvic bands and back supports, or sometimes spinal brace. As they progress, the back supports are removed, then the pelvic band and finally they wear below-knee irons. The full length brace has locking joints at hip and knee so that control can be taught with them locked or unlocked.

Muscle education Spastics are given muscle education based on an analysis of whether muscles are spastic, weak, normal or 'zero cerebral', or atonic. Muscles antagonistic to spastic muscles are activated. This is to obtain muscle balance between spastic muscles and their weak antagonists. Athetoids are trained to control simple joint motion and do not have muscle education. Ataxics may be given strengthening exercises for weak muscle groups.

Others, including Deaver [31], Pohl [32], Plum [33], Rood [35], Tardieu [36–37], have developed ideas on bracing and muscle education. Deaver uses braces for ambulation, eliminating brace elements as the child's control improves. He concentrates on self-care or activities of daily living, particularly the independent use of wheelchairs. Pohl focusses the child's attention on individual muscles for training a movement. Progress is made to movements of the limb and body. Plum advocates strengthening spastic muscles as well as their antagonists. However, he exercises the spastic muscles in their outer ranges as the muscles are usually shortened, whereas the antagonists are exercised in their middle and inner ranges. Tardieu, in a 'factorial analysis' identifies the specific problem in the muscles which gives rise to abnormal movements or deformities. According to this careful analysis, treatment is given where indicated. Alcohol injections are used to diminish spasticity, muscle education, specific bracing and a preference for early orthopaedic surgery are recommended. Unlike most of the other orthopaedic approaches, Tardieu's includes neurodevelopmental studies.

PROGRESSIVE PATTERN MOVEMENTS

Temple Fay [38–41], a neurosurgeon in Philadelphia, recommends that the cerebral palsied be taught motion according to its development in evolution. He regards ontogenetic development (in man) as a recapitulation of phylogenetic development (in the evolution of the species). In general, he suggests building up motion from reptilian squirming to amphibian creeping, through mammalian reciprocal motion 'on all fours' to the primate erect walking. As lower animals carried out these early movements of progression with a simple nervous system, they can similarly be carried out in the human in the absence of a normal cerebral cortex. The midbrain, pons and medulla could be involved in the stimulation of primitive patterns of movement and primitive reflexes which activate the handicapped parts of the body. Fay also described 'unlocking reflexes' which reduce hypertonus. Based on these ideas, he developed *progressive pattern movements* which consist of five stages:

Stage 1   Prone lying. Head and trunk rotation from side to side.

Stage 2   Homolateral stage. Prone lying, head turned to side. Arm on the face side in abduction-external-rotation, elbow semiflexed, hand open thumb out towards the mouth. Leg on face side in abduction, knee flexion opposite stomach, foot dorsiflexion. Arm on the occiput side is extended, internally rotated, hand open at the side of the child or on the lumbar area of his back. Leg on the occiput side is extended. Movement involves head turning from side to side with the face, arm and leg sweeping down to the extended position and the opposite occiput arm and leg flexing up to the position near the face as the head turns round.

Stage 3   Contralateral stage. Prone lying. Head turned to side, arm on the face side as in stage 2. The leg on the face side is, however, extended. The other leg on the side of the occiput is flexed. As the head turns this contralateral pattern changes from side to side.

Stage 4 On hands and knees. Reciprocal crawling and on hands and feet stepping in the 'bear walk' or 'elephant walk'.

Stage 5 Walking pattern. This is a 'sailor's walk' called by Fay 'reciprocal progression on lower extremities synchronised with the contralateral swing of the arms and trunk'. A wide base is used and the child flexes one hip and knee into external rotation and then places his foot on the ground, still in external rotation. As the foot is being placed on the ground, the opposite arm and shoulder are rotating towards it. As weight is taken on the straight leg, the other leg flexes up.

The Doman-Delacato system, which follows the basic tenets postulated by Fay, also recommends periods of inhalations of CO_2 from a breathing sack, restriction of fluid intake and development of cerebral hemispheric dominance. Cerebral dominance is attempted by principal use of dominant eye, hand, foot and arm and other methods. Children are also hung upside down and whirled around to stimulate the vestibular apparatus. They are also asked to hang and 'walk' their hands along a horizontal ladder as observed in apes.

The progressive pattern movements are first practised passively for 5 minute periods at least five times daily. One person turns the head, another person moves the arms and leg on one side, and another person the arm and leg on the other side. Locomotion beyond the stage of the child's patterning level is not permitted. A child who is not proficient in cross pattern creeping is prevented from walking. 'Neurological organisation' is considered possible if each developmental level is established before going to the next level.

SYNERGISTIC MOVEMENT PATTERNS

Signe Brunnstrom [42, 43], a physical therapist, produces motion by provoking primitive movement patterns or synergistic movement patterns which are observed in fetal life or immediately after pyramidal tract damage. The main features of her work are:

Reflex responses are used initially and later voluntary control of these reflex patterns is trained. Most of Brunnstrom's therapy has been on adult hemiplegics—in relation to the studies on the stages of recovery of flexion and extension limb synergies leading ultimately to isolated motion.

Control of head and trunk is attempted with stimulation of attitudinal reflexes such as tonic neck reflexes, tonic lumbar reflexes, and tonic labyrinthine reflexes. This is followed by stimulation of righting reflexes and later balance training.

Associated reactions are used as well as '*hand reactions*' e.g. hyperextension of the thumb produces relaxation of the finger flexors.

Brunnstrom uses proprioceptive and other *sensory stimulation* in her training programmes for adult hemiplegics.

PROPRIOCEPTIVE NEUROMUSCULAR FACILITATIONS [44–47]

Herman Kabat, a neurophysiologist and psychiatrist in the USA, has discussed various neurophysiological mechanisms which could be used in therapeutic exercises. With Margaret Knott and Dorothy Voss, he developed a system of movement facilitation techniques and methods for the inhibition of hypertonus. The main features of these methods are the use of:

Movement patterns (called 'mass movement patterns') based on patterns observed within functional activities such as feeding, walking, playing tennis, golf or football. These patterns are spiral (rotational) and diagonal with a synergy of muscle groups. The movement patterns consist of the following components:
1 Flexion or extension.
2 Abduction or adduction.
3 Internal or external rotation.

Sensory (afferent) stimuli are skilfully applied to facilitate movement. Stimuli used are touch and pressure, traction and compression, stretch, the proprioceptive effect of muscles contracting against resistance and auditory and visual stimuli.

Resistance to motion is used to facilitate the action of the muscles which form the components of the movement patterns.

Special techniques
1 *Irradiation*—this is the predictable overflow of action from one muscle group to another within a synergy or movement pattern or by *reinforcement* of action of one part of the body stimulating action in another part of the body.
2 *Rhythmic* stabilisations which use stimuli alternating from the agonist to its antagonist in isometric muscle work.
3 *Stimulation of reflexes* such as the mass flexion or extension.
4 *Repeated contractions* of one pattern using any joint as a pivot.
5 *Reversals* from one pattern to its antagonist and other reversals based on the physiological principle of successive induction.
6 *Relaxation* techniques such as contract-relax and hold-relax. Ice treatments are used for relaxation of hypertonus.
There are various combinations of techniques.

Functional work or 'mat work' involves the use of various methods mentioned above in training rolling, creeping, crawling, walking and various balance positions of sitting, kneeling and standing.

NEUROMOTOR DEVELOPMENT

Eirene Collis [2, 48], a therapist and pioneer in cerebral palsy in Britain stressed neuromotor development as a basis for assessment and treatment. Her main points were:

The mental capacity of the child would determine the results.

Early treatment was advocated.

Management—the word 'treatment' was considered misleading in that beside the physiotherapy session there should be 'management' of the child throughout the day. The feeding, dressing, toiletting and other activities of the day should be planned.

Strict developmental sequence—the child was not permitted to use motor skills beyond his level of development. If the child was, say, learning to roll he was not allowed to crawl, or if crawling he was not allowed to walk. At all times the child was given a 'picture of normal movement' and, as posture and tone are interwoven, Collis placed the child in 'normal postures' in order to stimulate 'normal tone'. Once postural security was obtained, achievements were facilitated and developmental sequences were followed throughout this training.

The C.P. Therapist Collis disliked the separation of treatment into physiotherapy, occupational therapy and speech therapy. She established the idea of the 'cerebral palsy therapist'.

NEURODEVELOPMENTAL TREATMENT WITH REFLEX INHIBITION AND FACILITATION

Karl Bobath, a neuropsychiatrist, and Berta Bobath [13–17, 49–52], a physiotherapist, base assessment and treatment on the premise that the fundamental difficulty in cerebral palsy is lack of inhibition of reflex patterns of posture and movement. The Bobaths associate these abnormal patterns with abnormal tone due to overaction of tonic reflex activity. These tonic reflexes, such as the tonic labyrinthine reflex, symmetrical tonic neck reflexes and asymmetrical tonic neck reflexes, have to be inhibited. In addition, various primitive reflexes of infancy should also be inhibited. Once the abnormal tone and reflex patterns have been inhibited, there should be facilitation of more mature postural reflexes. All this is carried out in a developmental context. The main features of their work are:

'*Reflex inhibitory patterns*' specifically selected to inhibit abnormal tone associated with abnormal movement patterns and abnormal posture.

Sensory motor experience   The reversal or 'break down' of these abnormalities gives the child the sensation of more normal tone and movements. This sensory experience is believed to 'feedback' and guide more normal motion. Sensory stimuli are also used for inhibition and facilitation and voluntary movement.

Facilitation techniques for mature postural reflexes.

'*Key points of control*' are used by the therapist for inhibition or facilitation.

Developmental sequence is followed and adapted to each child.

All day management should supplement treatment sessions. Parents and others are advised on daily management and trained to treat the children. Nancie Finnie has written a book for parents on this all-day handling of the child in the home [11].

SENSORY STIMULATION FOR ACTIVATION AND INHIBITION [35]

Margaret Rood [53–57], a physiotherapist and occupational therapist, bases her approach on many neurophysiological theories and experiments. The main features of her approach are:

Afferent stimuli   The various nerves and sensory receptors are described and classified into types, location, effect, response, distribution and indication. Techniques of stimulation, such as—stroking, brushing, (tactile)—icing, heating, (temperature)—pressure, bone pounding, slow and quick muscle stretch, joint retraction and approximation, muscle contractions (proprioception) are used to activate, facilitate or inhibit motor response.

Muscles are classified according to various physiological data, including whether they are for 'light work muscle action' or 'heavy work muscle action'. The appropriate stimuli for their actions are suggested.

Reflexes other than the above are used in therapy, e.g. tonic labyrinthine reflexes, tonic neck, vestibular reflexes, withdrawal patterns.

Ontogenetic developmental sequence is outlined and strictly followed in the application of stimuli.

1 Total flexion or withdrawal pattern (in spine).
2 Roll over (flexion of arm and leg on the same side and roll over).
3 Pivot prone (prone with hyperextension of head, trunk and legs).
4 Co-contraction neck (prone head over edge for co-contraction of vertebral muscles).
5 On elbows (prone and push backwards).
6 All fours (static, weight shift and crawl).
7 Standing upright (static, weight shifts).
8 Walking (stance, push off, pick up, heel strike).

Vital functions A developmental sequence of respiration, sucking, swallowing, phonation, chewing and speech is followed. Techniques of brushing, icing, pressure are used.

REFLEX CREEPING AND OTHER REFLEX REACTIONS

Vaslav Vojta [58–59], a neurologist working in Czechoslovakia, now in Germany, developed his approach from the work of Temple Fay and Kabat. The main features are:

Reflex creeping The creeping patterns involving head, trunk and limbs are facilitated at various 'trigger' points or 'reflex zones'. The creeping is an active response to the appropriate 'triggering' from the zones with sensory stimuli. The muscle work used in the normal creeping patterns or 'creeping complex' have been carefully analysed. The therapist must be skilful in the facilitation of these normal patterns and not provoke 'pathological patterns'.

Reflex rollings are also used with special methods of 'triggering'.

Sensory stimulation Touch, pressure, stretch and muscle action against resistance are used in many of the triggering mechanisms or in facilitation of creeping.

Resistance is recommended for action of muscles. Various specific techniques are used to apply the resistance so that either a tonic or a phasic muscle action is provoked. The phasic action (through range) may be provoked on, say, a movement of a limb creeping up or downwards. The tonic action, or stabilising action, is obtained if a phasic movement is prevented by full resistance given by the therapist. Therefore the static muscle action of stability occurs if resistance is applied so that it prevents any movement through range. *Rising reactions* are also provoked using resistance and all the methods above.

CONDUCTIVE EDUCATION [61–66]

Andras Petö in Budapest, Hungary, originated *conductive education*. Since Professor Petö's death, the work has been continued by Dr M. Hari [60]. The main features are:
The integration of therapy and education by having:

A conductor acting as mother, nurse, teacher and therapist. She is specially trained in the habilitation of motor disabled children in a 4-year course. She may have one or two assistants.

The group of children, about fifteen to twenty, work together. Groups are fundamental in this training system.

An all-day programme   A fixed time-table is planned to include getting out of bed in the morning, dressing, feeding, toiletting, movement training, speech, reading, writing and other schoolwork.

The movements   Sessions of movements take place mainly on and beside slatted plinths (table/beds) and with ladder-backed chairs. The movements are devised in such a way that they form the elements of a task or motor skill. The tasks are carefully analysed for each group of children. The tasks are the activities of daily living, motor skills including hand function, balance and locomotion. The purpose of each movement is explained to the children. The movements are repeated, not only in the movement sessions of, say the 'hand class' or 'plinth work', but also in various contexts throughout the day. The children are shown in practice how their 'exercises' contribute to daily activities.

Rhythmic intention   The technique used for training the elements or movements is 'rhythmic intention'. The conductor and the children state the intended motion: 'I touch my mouth with my hands'. This motion is then attempted together with their slow, rhythmic counts of one to five. Motion is also carried out to an operative word, such as 'up, up, up' repeated in a rhythm slow enough for the children's active movement ability. Speech and active motion reinforce each other.

Individual sessions may be used for some children to help them to participate more adequately in the work of the group.

Learning principles are basic to the programme. Conditioning techniques and group dynamics are among the mechanisms of training discussed. 'Cortical' or conscious participation is stressed, as opposed to involuntary and unconscious reflex therapy.

CHAPTER 4

SYNTHESIS OF
TREATMENT SYSTEMS

All the various treatment systems claim good results. It is difficult to decide which approach is superior whether on the basis of a scientific study or on theoretical grounds. Clinical experience of many therapists, as well as my own, has not confirmed the superiority of any one approach [67–76, 82].

A SCIENTIFIC STUDY

This is fraught with many problems and to date no study to compare the value of different treatment systems has convincingly dealt with all the problems. Firstly, the results of treatment of the motor handicap are influenced not only by the methods used, but also by the child's personality or 'drive' intelligence and home background as well as by the many possible associated handicaps of hearing, vision, perception or communication and by the presence of epilepsy. Matching children, apart from acquiring untreated controls, is difficult. One must also recognise that the enthusiasm, personality and skill of the therapist, rather than the particular system she is using, may have a strong effect on the results of treatment.

It is also difficult to compare systems of treatment by the records of the results achieved. The methods of assessment are often self-validating in terms of the theories of each system. Because the theories or concepts are controversial, such assessment of progress is not objective enough. In addition, therapists state the practical aims of particular methods in different ways. Achievement of any of these aims may be a 'good result' but may not make a great difference to the child's life. The superiority of different treatments cannot be assessed on the basis of these criteria. Any scientific study has to devise independent, valid and objective assessment techniques, as well as control the many variables and obtain untreated controls.

There are other problems. The results of a scientific study would have to be obtained over a long period of time. Crothers [71] pointed out many years ago that one would really need a long-term follow-up to adulthood to establish the ultimate effects of treatment methods in childhood.

THEORETICAL GROUNDS

Theoretical grounds for the different approaches depend on an understanding of brain function. This is highly controversial and cannot yet form a basis for the selection of the best treatment system. Every therapist wishes to understand 'why we do what we do' and, unfortunately, may accept a system because it offers a ready explanation. However, there is no all-encompassing theory that fully explains all the abnormal motor behaviour presented by the children, or the effects of various treatment procedures. Every system offers unproven neurophysiological and psychological hypotheses as well as reference to physiological experiments. Neuropsychology has rarely been used as a basis for treatment. Often normal physiology and normal child psychology are presumed to pertain to abnormal children. Is this necessarily so? And are the existing neurophysiological techniques subtle enough to bring about all the changes in the damaged nervous system that the theories claim?

Although the therapist should continue to ask herself why she is using a particular method, this enquiry should be focussed on the observation of the behaviour of abnormal children and any changes in behaviour after treatment procedures. The reason for using a technique should not rest on theoretical hypotheses of brain function at this stage of our knowledge. We have to learn to live with that doubt.

CLINICAL EXPERIENCE

This has shown that choice of methods for an individual child depends on age, sex, personality and level of motor development. Developmental levels in other areas such as vision, hearing, communication, understanding and perception influence selection of techniques. Consideration has also to be given to facilities for treatment, the training of existing therapists, and the part played by the parents and the community, as to which methods are practical. If the therapist wishes to help as many children as possible, she must increase her repertoire of methods and not confine herself to the methods she has obtained in one system [71–75, 87–90]. Some of these methods cannot be learnt without long instruction in a special course on the system in which these methods occur. However, there are methods in every system which do not require the full specialised course in order to learn them. Someone who is trained in any system can select techniques from that system and teach them to a qualified physiotherapist. But, unfortunately, this does not happen as someone following a system often cannot divorce her techniques from the total system.

In the synthesis of treatment systems, I have offered principles of treatment which make it possible to select techniques from different systems according to the individual behaviour of the child. The techniques can be carried out by a qualified physiotherapist, although it is always preferable that she be supervised by senior colleagues and attend a course with an eclectic approach. Those directing these courses must themselves have studied many different systems and know what to select from them according to the aptitudes of the students.

THE ECLECTIC VIEWPOINT IN THERAPY

As it is difficult to confine oneself to any particular system and as each has made valuable contributions, an eclectic approach is recommended. In developing the eclectic approach, it has been necessary to try to understand the rationale underlying the methods in various systems of treatment.

At first, the systems appear different and even contradictory to one another. However, this is not really the case. Although there are differences, there is also common ground. The following discoveries emerged in my comparative study of the theory and practice of various treatment approaches:

1   Different rationale are given by different systems for the same or similar methods. The common ground is the method, but the reasons offered differ.
2   In some instances, the rationale are not really different, but only couched in different terminologies. The common ground is both the method and the reason for it.
3   In other instances, the rationale are the same, only couched in different terminologies, but the methods suggested differ from system to system. The common ground is the rationale but methods differ.
4   There are still differences in methods and rationale.
5   Although methods may differ they are sometimes given the same name.

I have attempted to analyse and clarify this complicated field in order to bring together isolated, but valuable pockets of knowledge. During these studies, it has also been difficult to know which methods and ideas in any particular system are the ones which are responsible for the results achieved. In any system there are methods and ideas which are superfluous. It is not correct that 'everything in a system depends on everything else.'

Methods and ideas have been selected rather more according to the problems of the children than according to the theories underlying the methods. In this way a synthesis of treatment can be made.

SYNTHESIS OF TREATMENT SYSTEMS

Despite different terminologies and methods the following aspects are fundamental to the various systems of treatment.
1   The postural mechanisms.
2   Voluntary motion.
3   Perceptual motor function.

THE POSTURAL MECHANISMS

Purdon Martin [30] has studied and described the various postural mechanisms in a clear and practical way. I have found his particular presentation useful in clarifying the terminologies and methods in different approaches. His classification can also be used by the therapist in drawing on the various treatment approaches. In this book, it has been slightly modified and related to the problems of cerebral palsied children and other children who have motor delay.

The postural mechanisms are given and illustrated in the practical chapters 5, 6 and 8. In outline they consist of:

The antigravity mechanism or the mechanism which helps to support the weight of the body against gravity.

This is also known as the 'supporting reaction' in infants, 'leg straightening reflex' or 'positive statzreaktion'.

The postural fixation of parts of the body, i.e. head on trunk, trunk on pelvis and fixation of the shoulder girdles and pelvic girdles and the lower jaw, pharynx and tongue. Postural fixation of the body as a whole.

Terminologies also used for this are 'stability', 'heavy work', 'tonic activity'.

Counterpoising mechanisms are associated with postural fixation. They are adjustments of the trunk and other parts of the body so that a movement can be made whilst the person maintains posture or equilibrium. Movements of the limbs or head provoke these adjustments of equilibrium.

Terminologies also used are 'balance during motion', 'weight shifts', 'sway' and various 'balance exercises' and 'movement superimposed on co-contraction'.

Righting or rising reactions, make it possible for the person to rise from lying to standing, or sitting to standing or many other changes of position. Rising into position as well as returning to the original position are both part of these reactions. Other terminologies used are 'assumption of posture', 'moving into position' and 'movement patterns'. The latter is confusing as there are also movement patterns which are voluntary movements and different to these automatic changes of posture. 'Righting' is also used meaning either 'sway' or 'tilt' reactions and is not the sense in which I use it.

Tilt reaction when a person is tilted well off the horizontal plane and he adjusts his trunk so that he preserves his balance.

Reactions to falling or saving from falling   These are various reactions in the limbs which prevent the person from falling over, if the tilt reactions cannot preserve balance. These reactions do not, on their own, stop falling over completely. For example, the arms may be thrown out to save the person from falling forward, sideways, backwards and in more complicated patterns. If the person is falling over from the standing position he may stagger, hop or quickly place a foot out to stop the fall. In sitting, kneeling and other positions the legs also move in order to save the person from falling from these positions.

Other terminologies for these reactions are 'protective responses'. Particular arm saving reactions are also called 'parachute reactions', 'saving and propping on the hands', 'protective extension', 'arm balance responses', 'precipitation reaction' or 'head protective response'.

'Equilibrium reactions' or 'balance reactions' are also terms used which mean a combination of tilt and the limb reactions. These terms are confusing as *all* the postural reactions above are involved with equilibrium or balance. Maintaining a posture is synonymous with maintaining balance. Also, lack of tilt reaction seems to augment limb saving reactions and vice versa. This is seen in ataxic and athetoid children (pp. 9, 144).

Whatever the terminologies and different viewpoints, these postural reactions are stimulated or trained within all systems of therapy. However, particular systems have emphasised some, but not all of these neurological mechanisms. Therefore it is important to draw on all systems to make sure that none of the child's postural mechanisms are neglected. In addition, those systems that have given attention to all these problems have not necessarily suggested methods to cover the needs of all children and once again selection of methods is essential when children do not respond.

Besides the six main postural reactions above, there are also:

Locomotive reactions which serve to initiate stepping, continue stepping and stop stepping.

Ocular postural reflexes and also control of facial musculature are also interwoven with the postural mechanisms.

These reactions can be stimulated within Developmental Training, using methods drawn from different systems of treatment. It is helpful to follow motor developmental levels, for as the child acquires the motor abilities in these sequences, he is acquiring these neurological mechanisms. However, the sequences may vary in normal and abnormal children. This is discussed below in the section on Developmental Training.

VOLUNTARY MOTION

Voluntary motion which is purposeful, conscious, willed motion is sometimes confused with the active automatic movements which occur in the postural mechanisms such as rising or saving from falling. Although some of the automatic movement synergies are also seen in voluntary movement, stimulation of the automatic patterns only corrects abnormal postures and movements but does not contribute enough to the training of voluntary motion. Voluntary motion uses many different synergies and there may be a great variety of synergies in any one child for the same task. In time he chooses the most effective pattern. Voluntary motion is also bound up with postural mechanisms in that they help to create stable posture so that limbs can be accurately used. Arm function and hand movements require postural fixation and counterpoising of the trunk, and the shoulder girdle for coordination. Postural fixation and counterpoising of the head also helps eye–hand coordination.

Voluntary motion is, however, far more complex, in that it is involved with perceptual, praxic and cognitive function. Physiotherapists contribute neuromuscular techniques which include more than the stimulation of automatic arm and leg patterns of postural reactions. These patterns are drawn from many systems of treatment and are discussed in particular reference to arm and hand function in Chapter 6. Additional advice must be obtained from other disciplines working on the learning of motor skills, i.e. psychology, special education and physical education.

PERCEPTUAL MOTOR FUNCTION

The therapy systems explored in this book touch on the role of the physiotherapist, occupational therapist and speech therapist's contributions to stimulation of all the senses, linking of sensations, sensory discrimination, developing body image, body scheme, spatial relationships and direction and other aspects which are related to perceptual motor function. The psychologist, teacher and other specialists make specific structured contributions to these aspects. The neuromuscular techniques in the various therapy systems may be integrated with the perceptual motor training [106–112].

TREATMENT PRINCIPLES FOR A SYNTHESIS OF THERAPY SYSTEMS

The common ground between the different systems forms the principles of treatment. These common denominators will be discussed so that the therapist can understand where they exist and where differences are apparent or real.

General Principles of Treatment which are commonly accepted by various schools of thought have already been presented in Chapters 1 and 2 and are:
1 Team work.
2 Early treatment.
3 Repetition of a motor activity, whether it is neuromuscular techniques in treatment sessions or in the motor activity during all day management.
4 Sensory motor experience.
5 Motivation of the child.

Specific Principles of Treatment   Common factors detected in the various systems of treatment are:

1   Developmental training.
2   Treatment of abnormal tone.
3   Training of movement patterns.
4   Use of afferent stimuli.
5   Use of active movement.
6   Facilitation, abnormal and normal 'overflow'.
7   Prevention of deformity.

DEVELOPMENTAL TRAINING

Most systems of treatment suggest following the normal motor developmental sequences of child development. It is, however, superficial to advise therapists, as is frequently done, 'to follow normal motor developmental sequences'. Viewpoints differ as to whether to strictly follow these sequences, or modify them. Viewpoints also differ as to whether to train a total motor function such as rolling, crawling, standing or walking [6, 77] or whether to break each function down into elements for training [76, 17, 66, 53]. Most therapists prefer to train elements or 'bricks' which build up the motor function as well as train the total function [58]. However, views differ as to what these elements are. Some talk of different types of muscle tone, different reflexes, different muscle work and other ideas. In addition, 'basic motor patterns' are recommended as the basic abilities which underlie many motor functions on the developmental scales. For example, Bobath [17] suggests training the fundamental motor patterns of head and trunk control, symmetry, extensor activity, rotation, arm support and equilibrium reactions. Rood [53] suggests muscle work in main stages on an *Ontogenetic developmental sequence*, Vojta [58] uses the basic creeping complex from which stabilisation and rising are facilitated. Fay (Doman) [38–41, 68] uses levels of creeping, crawling and only prone development; Cotton [66] recommends symmetry, grasp, elbow extension, hip flexion and mobility as fundamental in cerebral palsy. It is possible to contain all these viewpoints in recognising that:

1   Training postural reactions and locomotive reactions described above, as well as movement patterns of voluntary motion, includes all these elements (see below). It is important to look at the postural reactions in each *part* of the body i.e. head, shoulder girdles, trunk, pelvic girdle and check at what level they are (Chapters 5 and 6).

2   Strict sequences are only relevant to the sequence of development of these postural reactions and voluntary motion and NOT to the sequence of milestones or *total* motor function. For example, it is easier for the child to acquire postural fixation of the head in a motor function at say 3 months normal developmental level than at say the more demanding functions at 6 and 9 months levels. Control of the head in supported sitting (3 months) is

easier than head and trunk control in unsupported sitting (7–9 months). Tilt reactions are easier in lying (6–9 months) than in sitting (9–12 months). Rising on to all fours (6–9 months) is easier than rising on to two feet (18 months).

3 Modifications of sequences are also needed for individual children to find their own pattern of development of the various postural reactions. For example, shoulder postural fixation and postural fixation of the head may be acquired not only when the child is in prone, leaning on forearms (at about the 3 months normal level), but also when he is sitting leaning on forearms on a low table, or standing leaning on forearms on a table. There are many examples of total motor functions at apparently higher levels on the developmental sequences that are useful in obtaining the same postural reactions which also occur in total motor functions at stages in earlier developmental milestones. The child may cope with such modifications of developmental sequences and *even require* them.

Omission of any motor function is not serious unless it also means the omission of a postural reaction. Therefore no child should be held back in order for him to acquire all the motor functions below and at his developmental level. Nor should the therapist 'go back' to fill in the gaps in his development unless these gaps are omissions of particular postural reactions or basic voluntary movement patterns.

4 Remember, postural reactions of one part of the body may be more advanced than another part, e.g. the head may be better than pelvis and vice versa; shoulder girdle may be better than pelvis and vice versa.

5 Modifications of the developmental sequences may also be required if a child has a preference for particular abnormal postures of the head, trunk or limbs. For example, repeated use of flexor postures and movements must be corrected by selection of motor functions which use more extension and any patterns *other* than the preferred flexion patterns.

6 Modifications of sequence are also indicated if a child strongly dislikes prone or other positions. Prone is commonly disliked in a few children who bottom shuffle rather than crawl before they walk, or in children with breathing problems. In addition, the full list of motor functions in prone development (or any other channel), may be impossible in hemiplegics or in others with severe involvement of both arms. It may still be possible to walk, to sit and to achieve the postural reactions and voluntary motion through other developmental motor functions [23].

Development ladder

As most systems of treatment consider that the elements of motor functions should be trained, and not only the total motor function, it is impossible to accept the view of using ONE developmental ladder.

The developmental training of the past trained first head control and only then rolling, next sitting, then crawling and only after all these standing and walking. This view may have arisen because these motor skills *appear* more or less in this sequence. However, in normal children all these skills are developing simultaneously but are not fully achieved until different milestones ('motor ages'; developmental levels) are reached. At birth, the child is able to take weight on his feet and momentarily hold his head upright. These are the elements of standing, but it will take many months before the full achievement of standing alone. The same occurs for crawling, for rolling and for sitting. The therapist should work on developmental sequences for each motor function or collection of functions in, say, supine, prone, sitting and standing positions. Parallel motor developmental channels are more relevant to therapy (Holt, Bobath, Levitt) [20, 17, 7].

To summarise This book uses parallel developmental sequences with selected motor activities which are fundamental postural reactions. In the practical chapters ideas are selected from various approaches to train the motor activities in the developmental sequences. Modifications of developmental sequences are recommended when necessary.

TREATMENT OF ABNORMAL TONE

Hypertonicity

Cerebral palsied children are often called spastics and to this day spasticity is given particular prominence in most systems of treatment. However, spasticity is not of great significance. If spasticity is reduced or even removed by, say, alcohol or phenol injections, the child will still be handicapped (Nathan [79]). Pederson [80] remarks on the lack of correlation of spasticity with voluntary motion in his review of alcohol and phenol injections. After removal of spasticity, the voluntary motion may be stronger, weaker or absent. Postural reactions are not correlated with spasticity. Observation shows that the emergence of postural reactions in developmental training will occur independently of whether the child is mildly or severely spastic. A spastic child may walk whereas a more mildly spastic may not do so. The degree of independent function depends on how developed their postural reactions become. Paine's studies [78] of the evolution of postural reflexes shows no correlation between them and increases or decreases of tone.

Purdon-Martin also found that his patients with Parkinson's disease showed no correlation between their rigidity and the presence of postural reactions [30]. The reason spastic children do not develop motor functions is not because of their spasticity. After all, at first spastic babies are often not spastic. However, they are motor handicapped as they do not have motor functions which depend on postural reactions [81].

There are situations when spasticity IS relevant to function. This is when spasticity contributes to abnormal postures or deformities which offer a mechanical block to function. As any experienced therapist knows, many deformities do not equal disability, or in other words do not always block function. Examples of blocking of function are plantarflexed feet which prevent the achievement of plantigrade feet needed for standing or in many cases as two extra props for helping to overcome insecure sitting; flexed knees in standing which prevents the postural fixation of the pelvis in the vertical position and the counterpoising mechanisms from operating efficiently for walking and for arm motion in standing; adductor spasticity which prevents a wide sitting base for the development of sitting.

Treatment of the spasticity varies from system to system. The neurophysiologists Eklund and Hagbarth have not been able to accept any of the theories as the 'answer' and support my suggestion that one should draw on different systems of treatment [82].

In all systems of treatment motor developmental levels of posture and movement are being trained. Thus the child is being helped to move as much as possible and this will *include* the treatment of the spasticity or other hypertonus. Treatment of the patterns of abnormal performance discussed in the practical chapters will counteract spasticity and deformities and help the child 'look better' as well as avoid any mechanical blocks to function.

See Chapter 8 for further discussion of spasticity in relation to deformity. This chapter shows that treatment of spasticity may be helpful, but in some cases removal of spasticity may even remove function if there are no normal postural reactions.

Remember, postural reactions are the normal postural reactions not the *abnormal* postural reflexes of tonic reflex activity (page 11).

Hypotonicity

Hypotonicity is also not correlated with strength of voluntary motion but seems more associated with the postural reactions. Improvement of the postural reactions seems to coincide with improvement of the hypotonic muscles (page 11). Tactile stimulation and other techniques aimed at increasing tone are useless unless accompanied by training of the motor functions or postural mechanisms, or in fact replaced by this training.

Fluctuating tone

Fluctuating tone or severe sudden spasms and involuntary motion seems to 'throw the child off balance', but may not prevent the development of the postural reactions. The association of these athetoid symptoms and postural reactions is not clear yet. Severe athetoids have disrupting spasms or tone fluctuations and severe disability in function. Nevertheless in some children voluntary motion can be trained, despite disturbance by the involuntary movements. Improvement of postural mechanisms seems to *decrease* the disrupting effect and sometimes the degree of involuntary motion.

To summarise The therapist should not collect techniques for abnormal tone *as such* but rather:

1 Emphasise training the motor functions composed of postural reactions and voluntary motion.

2 Enlarge the amount and variety of motor abilities.

3 Train the best pattern of performance so that deformity is prevented or decreased.

4 Concentrate on threatening and established deformities which may block function, e.g. spastic plantarflexors which contribute to toe standing and increase difficulty in sitting. A secure base is needed and provided by a pair of feet held flat on the ground.

The treatment of deformity involves many methods as well as orthopaedic surgery and the use of splintage, plasters and special equipment (see Chapter 8).

TRAINING OF MOVEMENT PATTERNS

Some therapy systems assess and treat individual muscle groups [26–33] (Phelps, Pohl, Plum) and this muscle education is associated with orthopaedics [83, 84]. Apparently contradictory views are held in the neurological approaches, which strongly recommend assessing and training movement patterns, and patterns of posture. There is no total contradiction for the following reasons.

1 Movement patterns are made up of muscle groups. In fact Tardieu points out that 'movement pattern' is a vague term as movement patterns may look the same, but be composed of different muscle actions in different children. Holt demonstrates with electromyography that the muscles acting in the same pattern of posture are different in different children. In orthopaedics, particular joints may be more deformed than others so that presumably some muscle groups are more troublesome than others *within* any abnormal patterns. It is therefore helpful to analyse the muscle-work in abnormal patterns of movements and posture [19, 20, 36, 37].

2 Although individual muscle groups may be assessed *in isolation* as is usual in orthopaedic physiotherapy, there is no need to follow such assessments with isolated muscle education. Muscle education can be obtained 'in pattern' as well. At low levels of development the child cannot easily isolate his movements. More severely brain damaged children and adults can only use mass movements or synergies of muscle action and cannot respond to localised muscle education.

3 Besides the level of function of any particular child, there is also the fact that training a muscle group, or relaxing a spastic muscle group, does not guarantee that the particular muscle group will work correctly within a function. Muscles are activated as prime movers, synergists or fixators when they contract, as well as being inhibited (relaxing, 'letting go') as

antagonists, during motion. Muscles have to shorten and contract (concentric work or isometric) keep the same length and contract (isotonic work) or lengthen and contract (eccentric work) in different movements. These various muscle actions are best trained in the movement in which they will be used. These movements are presented as various different movement patterns by different treatment systems. There are:

Movement patterns seen in the infantile reflex reactions (Table 5.2) such as the Moro, the Tonic neck, the withdrawal and crossed extension reactions and many others. There are also the primitive movements seen in normal infancy.

Movement patterns preferred by brain damaged patients which include normal primitive synergies such as the flexor synergy of hip flexion-knee flexion-dorsiflexion (the withdrawal reflex, mass flexion reflex, von Bechterew reflex or Strumpel's phenomena) or the extensor synergy of hip extension-knee extension-plantarflexion (extensor thrust), and crossed extensor reflex which is the flexor synergy in one leg with the extensor synergy in the other leg. There are also various abnormal patterns which are not primitive, in the sense that they may not be seen in normal infants, but which are only seen in neurological cases with damage to the central nervous system.

Mature patterns of movement seen in older children and adults. These patterns have more rotation and a variety of combinations of flexion and extension within any one synergy.

As the former two problems are indications of abnormality in children at 6 months of age and older, some therapists will not use these patterns in any children over 6 months. There are, however, children who are so immobile and severely handicapped that the primitive patterns are the only ones which are possible. The reflex creeping complex, reflex rolling, withdrawal reactions or automatic stepping may be used to provoke movement. Such movement is also selected to counteract persisting abnormal postures. A severe spastic may lie stiffly with his legs in extension-adduction-internal rotation. The legs will move into flexion-abduction-external rotation if reflex forward creeping is provoked. Fay called the reflex flexion and other reflex motion, 'unlocking reflexes' as they unlocked a spastic position or pattern. Snell, Perlstein, Brunnstrom and Phelps are some workers who found they could only achieve action of an inactive muscle group if this muscle group could be activated within these primitive synergies. Lack of action in particular muscle groups contributes to deformity and therefore these synergies variously termed 'mass reflexes', 'synkinetic motion', 'confused motion', 'primitive reflex patterns', were used [28, 42, 70].

It is, however, desirable to attempt more mature patterns if they are possible. These are for example the patterns of Kabat's 'mass movement patterns' seen in functional activities [44–47], and Bobath's mature patterns in the developing child [17, 18].

In the treatment of one child at one level of function, it would be contradictory to use methods for reflex movement patterns seen in brain damaged children or normal infants together with methods for mature synergies seen in normal young children or adults. The therapist uses only those techniques which relate to the level of development or capacity of any particular child's nervous system.

To summarise Considering the many different methods used for muscle education and movement pattern training, it is *generally* advisable to 'Stimulate movements initially through primitive mass patterns, reflexes (Fay, Kabat) confused motion (Phelps) or through synkinetic movements (Perlstein, Snell) then modify these primitive combinations of movements into more controlled and advanced patterns (Kabat, Bobath) and finally into selective or isolated movements (Phelps, Pohl, Plum among others)'. Hellebrandt summarises Coghill as saying 'that the earlier manifestations of movement are perfectly integrated total patterns within which partial patterns arise, acquiring various degrees of discreteness by a process of individuation' (Levitt [71]). The different patterns of movement in normal and abnormal motor development and the techniques of therapy for muscle work and movement pattern are discussed in the chapters on developmental training, and prevention and correction of deformity.

USE OF AFFERENT STIMULI: AUTOMATIC AND CONSCIOUS MOTOR ACTIVITY

Most treatment systems use afferent stimuli of touch, temperature (cutaneous) or pressure, stretch, resisted motion, joint compression or retraction (proprioceptive stimuli) as well as visual and auditory stimuli. With various methods, therapists use their hands on the child to elicit muscle actions, reduction of spasticity and stimulate movement patterns. These motor activities are often reflex responses, i.e. on an automatic level. The child 'reacts to the stimuli' and feels a movement or posture he cannot achieve himself. In time this sensory-motor experience helps him acquire the motion or posture on his own. The action of the muscles within the response of automatic movement or muscle action is 'active' as opposed to 'passive' motion. What is not active is the child's initiation of the motion or the child's active concentration or participation in carrying out the patterns of movement and postures. His active efforts are considered to increase spasticity or abnormal patterns of function (Bobath [52], Vojta [58]). Rood is quoted as saying 'let us use our heads to do other things than run our muscles [56].' It is emphasised that our muscle actions, movement synergies and postures are not carried out at a conscious level but on an involuntary, unconscious level. When we move and balance, we do not think of these actions.

It is important to recognise that movements and postures are involuntary AFTER they have been achieved. In the process of training motor function as, say, in learning to drive a car, play tennis or ice skate, concentration on the movement and equilibrium is needed. Children should concentrate on, say, directions for rising from the floor, on maintaining balance, on putting their hands out to save themselves, to stop themselves from falling during training. For example, blind children have been taught to save themselves with verbal instructions to 'put out their arms' (observed by Zinkin) [119]. Later this becomes automatic. Automatic reactions may be possible in some procedures and should also be provoked this way if it is possible.

The child should also have his conscious attention on the afferent stimuli used by the therapist, as they are often cues to direction or to parts of his body and convey what movement is required. In addition, the child can be asked to 'pull', 'push', 'stretch up', 'try to sit alone' and so on. Some children, especially younger and mentally low children, respond better to concentration on an incentive for a particular motion, 'touch this', 'catch this', and on the motivation of toys and play. Neurophysiological techniques to facilitate automatic motion and counteract abnormal motor activity has obviously to be interwoven with the child's conscious participation.

The Petö approach is particularly careful to use the child's 'cortical' or conscious control of motion [61–65]. However, this approach does not carry out every aspect of motion consciously. The active efforts may focus on, say, voluntary arm motion whilst automatic head and trunk control occur. Conscious actions that are selected do not aggravate spasticity as these active motor activities are not too far ahead of the child, so that he is 'pushed' to make abnormal efforts to achieve a movement. The afferent stimuli are contained in the auditory and visual stimuli in the instructions the children use. 'Fixation' of a part of the child's body may involve manual contact with the child. However, little of the training of motion is based on afferent stimuli by the therapist handling the child.

To summarise It is advisable to show the child how and where to move by the therapist's afferent stimulii for automatic movements and postures. However, as soon as possible and even in the same therapy session, check whether the child can carry out the motor activity on his own even though it will be partial or unreliable. He should then concentrate and practice the motor activity without being handled or touched by the therapist. The motor activity selected should be at his level of development so that he can achieve something on his own. The child gains more from any corrective motor activity that he does himself. If, however the child is so severely handicapped that there is no activity possible on his own, facilitation with afferent stimuli or handling may be the only way to begin motor activity.

PASSIVE OR ACTIVE MOTION

Zuck *et al.* [24] and others have shown that active movement obtained more progress than passive procedures of passive motion and bracing. Passive 'patterning' of children or a 'full range of passive motion' cannot contribute much if anything to training motion. They only keep the joints mobile, and help to prevent deformity.

Passive correction by splintage, plasters, orthopaedic surgery passively change the child's positions so that he obtains a better proprioceptive experience or position from which to develop active motor function. Passive correction of, say, the child's feet in plasters makes his active correction of knees and hips and balance possible (de Rijke [85]).

Passive motion may be used to show the child what motion is required, but afferent stimuli are more effective as the active response to these stimuli give a better proprioceptive as well as visual-auditory demonstration of what is required. Active or active resisted motion provide better proprioceptive information than passive motion (Kabat [46], Held [86]).

The section on automatic and conscious movement (page 43) should also be read to obtain the whole picture of the controversy of Active and Passive therapy.

FACILITATION, ABNORMAL AND NORMAL 'OVERFLOW'

Many systems of treatment have used the activation of one part of the body to facilitate action in another part of the body, e.g. arm elevation simultaneously activates head elevation and back extension, creeping techniques triggered at the legs facilitate activity in the whole child. Stimulation of one part of a synergic movement pattern activates the other muscle groups within the same synergy. These facilitation techniques involve normal 'overflow' of activity from one area of the body to another.

It is however possible to activate undesirable actions in other parts of the body, e.g. grasping may increase flexion in the elbows and shoulders in a child already round-shouldered and flexed, use of the arms may increase spastic abnormal postures in the legs and grasping with one hand may be associated with clenching of the other hand. There are other abnormal 'associated reactions' observed by Bobath. Repetition of such abnormal 'overflow', as opposed to the normal 'overflow' of facilitation techniques, may aggravate abnormal postures and increase deformities. Facilitation techniques, including afferent stimuli and the use of resisted motion, must be used in such a way that the rest of the body does not become abnormal (Levitt [87–90]).

In this context it is important to combine the ideas of Bobath with those of Knott in facilitating motion. Knott facilitates motion in one part of the body with afferent stimuli and resistance. The rest of the body must be 'positioned' so that abnormal 'overflow' does not occur. Vojta's techniques uses resistance to creeping but, as the whole body is moving in a corrective pattern, 'positioning' is unnecessary. Also much rotation within facilitation patterns in spastics prevents 'overflow' of spasticity to other parts of the body.

To summarise   Any patterns facilitated in one part of the body should be accompanied by careful observation of the whole child and not only of the part being activated. Normal or abnormal 'overflow' of motor activity should be observed when using techniques in one part of the body to facilitate activity in other parts of the body.

PREVENTION OF DEFORMITY

Every system aims to prevent or correct deformity. There are many methods to counteract deformity as well as many viewpoints as to the genesis of deformity. Chapter 8 is devoted to this aspect.

CHAPTER 5

ASSESSMENT FOR
THERAPY AND DAILY CARE

In Chapters 1 and 2 on the principles and organisation of treatment it is obvious that the therapist requires a comprehensive assessment as well as her own specific assessment to understand why the child is delayed and has a motor disorder. The total and specific assessments are used:

To plan a therapy programme which includes special neuromuscular techniques, selection of equipment and advice to parents and others caring for the child.

To assess progress which may lead to continuation, modification, changes or sometimes periodical stopping of specific therapy sessions.

To add observations to the diagnostic picture. The therapist should also add to the diagnostic information as her specific assessments before *and* during therapy involves long periods of time and close contact with the child and his family. Information may be revealed to the therapist which may not have been obvious in the shorter consultations with the different consultants. General behaviour as well as specific problems should be observed by therapists [91, 92, 93].

ASSESSMENT METHODS

These vary from Centre to Centre and work is still in progress to find universal assessments which are objective, reliable, valid and relevant to practical therapy. Assessment methods have been reviewed elsewhere (Kendall [97], Holt [98], Levitt [99], Wolff [100]) and studies of these are being made (Durukan [101]).

This chapter offers a framework for assessment for practical therapy. As a synthesis of various systems is used in therapy it is not possible to use assessment methods from any one approach. However, the common factor in all treatment systems is that they all ultimately aim at the child's independent motor function. Therefore a functional assessment is used. (Chart, pp. 242–243). In addition all systems aim to prevent and counteract deformity and so an assessment of deformity is also required.

It is hoped that the assessment framework offered in this Chapter should show the therapist that assessment is directly involved with therapy.

If assessment does *not* do this, it will not be surprising that the therapist 'does not have time to assess'.

THE FUNCTIONAL ASSESSMENT

It is not enough to examine whether the child can carry out a list of motor functions. The developmental levels of these functions in normal children should be known so that the therapist can appreciate the degree of retardation in the child. In this way she will also understand how the motor delay may influence function in other areas of development.

If a developmental sequence for the motor function is carefully selected, it can be used not only for assessment but as a general guideline for therapy.

Developmental levels—assessment and therapy

The therapist should examine the child in the parallel developmental channels for prone development, supine development, sitting development standing and walking development (Chart, pp. 242–243) and development of hand function (Table 6.1, p. 185).

She should find out: *What the child can do; what the child cannot do* and *the way in which the child moves*

What the child can do These abilities will be equivalent to those in a normal child at a '*normal motor developmental level*' given in the practical chapters on each channel of development.

1 Begin therapy at the next stage on the channel of development.

2 Also attempt items at higher levels at the same time IF there is an ACTIVE flicker of response in the child at those levels.

3 Always check that the way in which the child carries out his present achievement is in as good a pattern as possible before concentrating on the higher levels of development.

What the child cannot do These abilities will be found at developmental levels above his achievement as well as gaps in his development below his levels of achievement. In the practical chapters these absent abilities are called '*delay in*'.

1 The higher levels have already been discussed above.

2 The gaps or omissions of items below the child's level may be of no significance or may account for the abnormal performance or for the inability to progress along the developmental channel being used by the child. Each child must be individually considered as it is illogical to train all items on developmental sequences in very handicapped children.

3 Ignore omissions of postures and movements if their postural reactions or voluntary movements can be trained in other or more advanced motor abilities.

4 Do not ignore omissions if this results in the child's repertoire of pos-

tures and movements being biassed towards certain recurring positions of his joints, e.g. predominance of flexion movements and flexion postures.

The way in which the child moves This is called 'abnormal performance' in the practical chapters that follow. Check that what the child can do is not being carried out in one of the common abnormal patterns described under abnormal performance or *any other* pattern which does not look similar to one seen in normal children at that particular level of function.

1   Correct the abnormal performance at the child's level of development.
2   Anticipate abnormal performances by checking on those possible at the next level of function and use methods to prevent them as much as possible.
3   Do not always insist on NORMAL patterns as this may be impossible in a child with a damaged nervous system. Attempt the best pattern possible.
4   Always try and find out whether the child can 'find his own' way of functioning independently if normal or near normal patterns are very difficult and frustrating for him and he is an older child.
5   Atypical pattern does not matter in the young child if they do not cause deformities. Athetoids are often those children who may achieve unexpected independence this way.

Grading

Grading of the child's achievements is essential for therapy, for advice to those who care for the child, and for recording progress. Grading a motor ability as 'beginning', 'partially achieved' and 'fully achieved' is in tune with the way both normal and abnormal children develop. The 'yes or no' grading will reveal no progress when the child has really achieved 'the beginning' of a new skill or 'partially achieved' it. In these cases therapists and parents have also found that with giving some additional assistance, these skills can be fully achieved by the child and ease the life of the child and the family. 'No progress' is not only inaccurate but discouraging to everyone in these slow developing children. Various gradings exist in different Centres. I do not use those that chart any assistance as this is difficult to measure, remember or record without long descriptions of *how much*, *where given* and *for how long* within the duration of the motor act. Assessment is primarily to find out how the child copes without any help. Assistance may be recorded as part of the advice for parents and others caring for the child. It is of course essential to 'record' this information in the minds of those caring for the child by demonstration.

Grading may be:

1   No ability.
2   Beginning, partially achieved, unreliable, insecure, momentary.
3   Reliably achieved, efficient.

It is obvious that the items on the developmental channels will be assessed and graded so that the therapist finds out what he cannot do (1) what he can do (2, 3). Grading 4 can include 'reliable with good pattern' as opposed to *very* abnormal pattern in 3. Abnormal performance or pattern is par-ticularly difficult to grade on a chart. It is, however, essential to have a grading or some record for therapy and for progress. A child may not only progress by obtaining a new ability but also by improving *the way* he carries out his existing abilities.

Therapists must observe the child's head, trunk, arms, legs in all motor activities during assessment and during therapy. Depending on the child and the therapist's experience much time may be needed.

This information may be written out or an attempt to grade this infor-mation may be made in general groups of severe, moderate and mild. This is possible if the categories are described in a list of instructions but it is seldom strictly accurate. If grading includes 'very abnormal' and 'good' therapists will be accurate in this more obvious range. There are other tools for observation and recording which include films, videotapes, various photographic methods, notation methods such as that of Benesh, Laban and others, electromyography and other more specific methods for specific problems of weight bearing, spasticity, joint range, gait pattern and so on [19, 20, 102–104].

ABNORMAL PERFORMANCE AND DEFORMITY

Observation of abnormal performance is the primary but not only obser-vation of abnormal positions of the joints in posture and movement. These are the unfixed or fixed deformities. Specific examinations of the child's joints and muscles should also be made to check whether there is a fixed or unfixed deformity. Fixed deformity due to structural change, leg length, or soft tissue contraction will explain abnormal performance on a mechani-cal level. Unfixed deformity is more complicated.

Examination of deformity

The therapist should obtain information on:

Structure of joints especially subdislocation or dislocation of the hips, varus or valgus neck of femur, spinal vertebrae.

Inequality in the length of legs but not so much in the arms, as far as func-tion is concerned.

Joint range   Passive range of motion carried out slowly may detect fixed or unfixed deformity as well as tightness of muscle groups. Quick passive stretch detects *hypertonus*. Active range is also needed but has already been observed in the functional examination where it is of the greatest significance.

Passive range (Figures and Captions—Table 5.1)

Table 5.1   Assessment of joint range

Assess:
Passive joint range: to demonstrate muscle length (extensibility, shortening), muscle tightness (spasticity, rigidity) and soft tissue tightness. Remember that muscle tightness (hypertonus) may or may not have full range of motion.
Degree of tightness or resistance to your passive motion, and where the greatest degree occurs in the range.
The difference between muscle and soft tissue tightness. Test *slowly*, use inhibitory techniques and sometimes anaesthetics to inhibit muscle tightness and reveal true contracture (fixed deformity).
Active joint range for range and ability to move and *not* as equivalent to muscle strength. Quality of muscle action should be noted. Strength and the opposing degree of tightness affect active range.
Note: Different positions may affect range of motion in some cases. Check in supine, prone, sitting, sidelying, standing as well.

Hip flexor tightness—extension range
Bend one knee to chest. The other may flex off bed. Overcome this hip flexion by downward pressure on the front of the thigh: Check how far this can be overcome, and how much pressure is required.

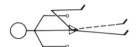

or
Bend both knees to chest. Hold one bent and see how far the other can be stretched down to the bed.
Prone-hip extension is usually inaccurate because of pelvic-truck compensation.

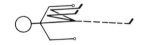

Hip extensor tightness—flexion range
Bend both hip and knee to chest. Note range and degree of extensor tightness. Hip extensor tightness also revealed in knee flexor test for hamstrings below.

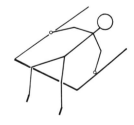

Hip adductor tightness—abduction range
Test in supine and in prone. Abduct hips with hips straight, knees bent. Abduct hips with hips and knees flexed. Abduct hips with hips and knees extended. These three procedures reveal tightness in different muscle groups and show which requires therapy and positioning. 50–80° is normal abduction with extended hips.

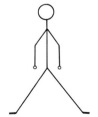

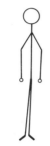

Hip adductor tightness—abduction range
Bring legs together and hips straight from 'frog position' if present.

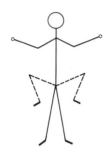

Hip rotator tightness—internal or external rotation
Assess with hip and knee flexed and extended. Rotate thigh inwards and outwards.

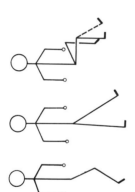

Knee flexor tightness—extension range
Bend one knee to eliminate hip flexion-lordosis and test the other. With hip at 90–100° fully extend that flexed knee.

Straight leg lift also reveals tight hamstrings (flexor tightness at knees and extensor tightness at hips).

Press knees straight in lying supine or prone (limited range may be detected).

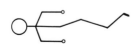

Knee extensor tightness—flexion range
Flex the knee. If hip rises up into flexion, press hip down as far as possible to detect tightness of biceps femoris.

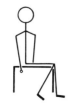

Sitting: flex knee for tightness of quadriceps.
Note any 'high-riding' patella.

Lying knees flexed over edge of bed without lordosis. Bend one knee to counter lordosis and also eliminate hip flexor tightness (if present) with tests above.

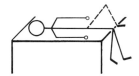

Foot plantar flexion tightness—dorsiflexion range
Bend hip and knee and dorsiflex foot by grasping heel and *avoiding* passive dorsiflexion in mid-foot. Hold dorsiflexion with knee straight.
Foot: inversion, eversion, plantarflexion tested with knee straight.

Note: keep pelvis level (stop A-P tilt, lateral tilt) during assessments

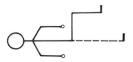

Shoulder flexor tightness—extensor range
Bring arm straight back.

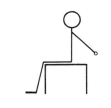

Shoulder flexor-adductor tightness—elevation range
Elevate arm forward and overhead.
Abduct and elevate arm.

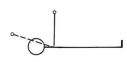

Shoulder rotations internal–external

Elbow flexor tightness—extension range
Slowly stretch *without* forcing elbow into extension with pronation and into extension with supination.

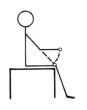

Elbow extensor tightness—flexion range
Bend elbow with pronation and test with supination.

Elbow pronation-supination
Carry out test with upper arm close to side of body.

Wrist flexion-extension

Wrist deviation radial and ulnar

Finger and thumb adduction and abduction

Finger and thumb flexion-extension
Remember to hold thumb at its base.

Head and trunk
Ranges rarely assessed unless torticollis or scoliosis is present.

Active ranges assessed as above but denotes action of antagonists overcoming tightness of agonists above. See also assessment within functional examinations.
Check: speed—rhythm—endurance of active assessments here and in functional assessments.
Note: Goniometry is measurement used for degrees of joint ranges.
Grade strength accurately as only: 'present' 'weak' 'strong'.

Active range (Table 5.1)

Head and Trunk flexion, extension, rotation observed during head raise in prone, supine, sitting developmental channels.

Shoulder elevation, abduction, rotation, flexion and extension movements are observed during the functional examination of, say, creeping, reaching and other arm movements.

Elbow flexion and extension observed during child's reach to parts of his body or toys. Forearm pronation or supination affects flexion and extension, and must also be seen in isolation.

Wrist and hand will be observed during hand function development.

Hip flexion and extension will be observed during all functions. Also ask the child to lie supine, bend his hip and knee to his chest and touch his feet and to sit and bend to touch the ground, to sit on very low stools and come up to standing and sit down again.

Knee flexion and extension seen with active hip flexion extension, as well as observing the child sitting using active extension to kick your hand or a dangling toy, and his knee extension in standing 'tall'.

Foot movements need to be tested separately especially if there are abnormal feet.

If the child cannot achieve a full active range check:
1 That it is not due to a decrease in the passive range of motion of the joint.
2 That it is not due to weakness, primary or secondary.
3 That it is not due to interference of abnormal reactions occurring during any particular activity.

The chapter on deformity should be read to understand the various possibilities for abnormal active joint range. Examination of isolated active joint range can only indicate that there is or is not activity in a muscle group but not whether that activity will occur in a function where it is really needed. Postoperative physiotherapy may occasionally require this localised assessment to confirm that muscle groups which have been given the opportunity to act by the operation are in fact doing so. They often are, but need strengthening due to disuse.

SPEED OF PERFORMANCE

Independence of a handicapped child is not fully achieved if he cannot move

Fig. 5.1   **Neurological reactions in development**

Based on: Illingworth, Paine, Bobath, Vojta, Prechtl, Milani, André-Thomas
Selected by: Sophie Levitt
Prepared by: Filiz Durukan   – For therapy techniques

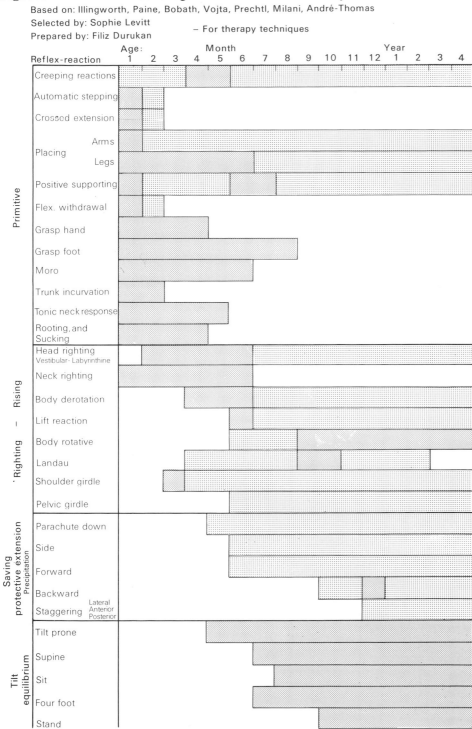

Table 5.2 Reflex reactions. A reflex conveys a stereotyped response to a stimulus. As responses vary in children the term reflex reaction is used.

Reflex reaction	Normal until	Stimulus	Response	Therapy
Sucking	3 months	Introduce a finger into mouth	Sucking action of lips and jaw	Train correct feeding
Rooting	3 months	Touch baby's cheek	Head turns toward stimulus	
Cardinal points	2 months	1 Touch corner of mouth	1 Bottom lip lowers on same side and tongue moves toward point of stimulation when finger slides away, the head turns to follow	Desensitive face by child's own touch and other stimuli by therapist
		2 Centre of upper lip is stimulated	2 Lip elevates, tongue moves toward place stimulated. If finger slides along oronasal grove the head extends	
		3 Centre of bottom lip is stroked	3 Lip is lowered and tongue directed to site of stimulation. If finger moves toward chin, the mandible is lowered and head flexes	
Grasp	3 months	Press finger or other suitable object into palm from ulnar side	Fingers flex and grip object. (Head in mid-line during this test)	Weight bearing, stimuli over whole hand, hand opening (see Development Hand Function, p. 169)
Hand opening	1 month	Stroke ulnar border of palm and little finger	Automatic opening of hand	
Foot grasp	9 months	Press sole of foot behind the toes	Grasping response of feet	Weight bearing (see Development of Standing, p. 149)
Placing	Remains	Bring the anterior aspect of foot or hand against the edge of a table	Child lifts limb up to step onto table	Use in provoking early step
Primary walking (Automatic Walk: Reflex Stepping)	2 months	Hold baby upright and tip forward, sole of foot presses against table	Initiates reciprocal flexion and extension of legs	Weight bearing (see Development of Standing, p. 149)
Galant's Trunk incurvation	2 months	Stroke back lateral to the spine	Flexion of trunk towards side of stimulus	Train trunk stability (see Development of Sitting and Standing (pp. 116–146)
Automatic sitting	2 months	Pressure is placed on the thighs and the head is held in flexion. Supine position.	Child pulls to sitting from supine	Train child's own rising (see Development of Sitting, p. 96)
Moro	0–6 months	Baby supine and back of head is supported above table. Drop head backwards, associated with loud noise	Abduction and extension of arms. Hands open. This phase is followed by adduction of the arms as if in an embrace	Train vertical head stability, use grasp, use prone position, use flexion position, shoulder fixation with grasp or hand support

Reflex reaction	Normal until	Stimulus	Response	Therapy
Startle	Remains	Obtained by sudden loud noise or tapping the sternum	Elbow is flexed (not extended as in the Moro reflex) and the hand remains closed	Desensitive to noise by warning and experience
Landau	From 3 months to 2½ years,	Child held in ventral suspension, lift head	The head, spine and legs extend. Extend arms at shoulders	Use in therapy to activate extensor muscles
	Strong 10 months	When the head is depressed	The hip, knees and elbows flex	
Flexor withdrawal	2 months	Supine; head mid-position, legs extended—stimulate sole of foot	Uncontrolled flexion response of stimulated leg (do not confuse with response to tickling)	⎫
Extensor thrust	2 months	Supine; head, mid-position, one leg extended, opposite leg flexed—stimulate sole of flexed leg	Uncontrolled extension of stimulated leg (do not confuse with response to tickling)	Weight bearing, Joint compression, Knee Splints and Calipers (see Development of Standing, p. 149)
Crossed extension	2 months	Supine; head, mid-position; legs extended—stimulate medial surface of one leg by tapping	Opposite leg adducts, extends internally rotates and foot plantarflexes (typical scissor position)	⎭
Asymmetrical tonic Neck (ATNR) reaction	Rare 6 months, usually pathological	Patient supine; head in mid-position; arms and legs extended—turn head to one side	Extension of arm and leg on face side, or increase in extensor tone; flexion of arm and leg on skull side or increase in flexor tone	Use both arms together and train head in midline, use prone position, only encourage in severe older child
Symmetrical tonic neck (STNR) neck reflex	Rare and usually pathological	1 Patient in quadruped position or over tester's knees—ventroflex the head	Arms flex or flexor tone dominates; legs extended or extensor tone dominates	(see Prone Development, p. 8) Correct weight bearing on hands and knees. If correct abnormal posture in all development then usually ignore the STNR
		2 Position as above, dorsiflex the head	Arms extend or extensor tone dominates; legs flex or flexor tone dominates	
Tonic labyrinthine supine	Pathological	Patient supine; head in mid position; arms and legs extended. Test stimulus—is the position	Extensor tone dominates when arms and legs are passively flexed	(see Development in Supine, p. 94); Development of Sitting, p. 111) Overcomes excessive extension
Tonic labyrinthine prone 'Reaction to prone'	3 months	Turn patient prone—head in mid position. Test stimulus—prone position	Unable to dorsiflex head, retract shoulders, extend trunk, arms, legs	(see Development in Prone, p. 70) Overcomes excessive flexion
Positive supporting	3 months	Hold patient in standing position—press down on soles of feet	Increase of extension in legs. Plantarflexion, genu recurvatum may occur	(see Development of Standing, p. 149) Excessive anti-gravity response
Negative supporting	3–5 months	Hold in weightbearing position	Child 'sinks' astasia	(see Development of Standing, p. 149)

Reflex reaction	*Normal until*	*Stimulus*	*Response*	*Therapy*
Neck righting	5 months	Supine, rotate head to one side, actively or passively	Body rotates as a whole in same direction as the head	(see Development of Rolling in Supine p. 98) Stimulate body rotative reactions
Associated reactions	Pathological	Have patient squeeze an object (with a hemiplegic, squeeze with uninvolved hand)	Clench of other hand or increase of tone in other parts of the body. Abnormal overflow	(see Development of Hand functions, p. 181)

Reflex reaction	*Emerges at*	*Stimulus*	*Response*	*Therapy*
Rising Labyrinthine head righting Vestibular righting (decrease of head lag)	2–6 months	1 Hold blindfolded patient in prone position, in space, as head drops	Head raises to normal position, face vertical, mouth horizontal	
		2 As above in supine position	Head raises to normal position, face vertical, mouth horizontal	
	6 months	3 Hold blindfolded patient in space—hold around pelvis tilt to the side	Head rights itself to normal position, face vertical, mouth horizontal	
Optical	6 months	AS ABOVE NO BLINDFOLD	AS ABOVE	
Amphibian	4–6 months	Patient prone, head in mid position, legs extended, lift pelvis on one side	Automatic flexion outward of hip and knee on same side	(see all Developmental training, pp. 70–169)
a Body righting derotative	4–6 months	Supine—rotate head or one knee one side, *passively*	Active derotation at waist, i.e. segmental rotation of trunk between shoulders and pelvis	
b Rotative	6–10 months	rotate hip and knee or arm or head *actively*	Active segmented rotation (hyperactive at 10 months cannot lie supine)	
Lift reaction (*not* the pathological 'lift reaction' (Tardien))	5–6 months	Lift body through space	Head raises (lifts)	
Shoulder/pelvic girdle righting	3–6 months	Fix distal part(s) of limb	rise up onto limb	

Postural fixation   (see Developmental Training, pp. 70–169)
counterpoising

Tilt reactions

a	Supine and prone	6 months	Patient on tiltboard. Arms and legs extended, tilt board to one side	Lateral curving of head and thorax, protective reaction in limbs accompany trunk reaction
b	Four point kneeling	7–12 months	Patient in quadruped position, tilt toward one side	Lateral curving of head and thorax. Abduction-extension of arm and leg on raised side and protective reactions on lowered side may accompany this
c			Tilt forward and back (A.P.)	Forward—Head and back, flex. Backward—Head and back, extend
d	Sitting	9–12 months	Patient seated on chair— tilt patient to one side Tilt forward antero-posterior back	Head and thorax curve abduction-extension of arm and leg on raised side, other protective reactions may accompany this
e	Sitting		Tilt forward	Child extends head and back
			Tilt back	Child flexes head and trunk
f	Kneel-standing	18 months	Patient in kneel-standing position, pull or tilt patient to one side	AS ABOVE
g	Standing	12–18 months	Patient in standing position. Tilt sideways. Tilt anteroposteriorly	TRUNK AS ABOVE

Staggering reactions	12–18 months	1	Move to left or to right side push or holding upper arm	Hopping, or step sideways to maintain equilibrium
(see Saving from Falling)		2	Move forward	Hopping, or step forwards to maintain equilibrium
		3	Move backwards	Hopping, or step backwards to maintain equilibrium or dorsiflex feet going on to heels
Saving from falling	5–10 months		Prone—sudden tip downward Sitting—sudden tip downward Standing—sudden tip downward	Immediate extension of arms with abduction and extension of fingers to to save and then prop the child
	6–9 months		Standing—sudden tip sideways—one arm	
	9–12 months		Standing—sudden tip backwards—both arms	

Note   Motor patterns of the responses may be abnormal

fast enough for his particular needs in his particular environment. To help
the children fit into normal schools or later normal work situations as well
as live with normal people in society they should be trained to function at
reasonable speed. This could be slower than normal but not *very* slow.
It is easy to assess when a child is very slow and therapy is adjusted accord-
ingly. Other speeds have to be assessed if they are relevant to the child's
life. Normal society can wait for the handicapped to keep up in many
situations.

REACTIONS RESPONSES AND REFLEXES

These should be known to the therapist so that she recognises them during
any motor functions on the developmental channels. These are summarised
in Tables and linked with therapy suggestions (pages 53–57). They should
not be examined by the therapist in isolation except as an academic exercise
or with the doctor for diagnostic information. Normal Postural reactions
are all assessed within the channels of development (Chapter 6).

VOLUNTARY MOTION

This is part of the assessment of the motor developmental channels (Chart)
and is specially observed in the development of arm and hand function, and
activities such as feeding and dressing. Arm or leg patterns in the postural
reactions of saving from falling and rising reactions are *not* the assessment
of limb patterns in voluntary or purposeful movement in play, feeding,
dressing and other activities.

ABNORMAL TONE

This is really considered when assessment is made of the abnormal performance. It should not be assessed as such but rather as 'tone' manifests itself
in the functions of the developmental abilities. The assessment of deformity
also includes assessment of the manifestation of abnormal tone. Assessment
of 'degree and distribution of tone' is superfluous as the degree does not
correlate with function, and distribution is obvious in the assessment of
motor delay and abnormal performance.

MUSCLE STRENGTH

This is only assessed after the assessment of the functional examination as
quite often it is no longer indicated then. The important observation is when
muscles act *in function* and whether this action is a holding action for

postural fixation or a moving action in voluntary motion or in rising, saving reactions or in stepping. The examination of deformity may have to include examinations of muscle strength. See active joint range (Table 5.1).

ADDITIONAL ASSESSMENT REQUIRED

Sensory examination Loss of sensation in the cerebral palsies is rare having only been described in hemiplegia (Tizard). Also it is difficult to assess sensation in babies and young, developmentally disabled children. Perceptual disorder or agnosias are much more common and various assessments are available and best done by neurologists, psychologists and specialised occupational therapists and teachers. Lack of body awareness and other perceptual problems may be lack, rather than loss, of *sensory experience.*

Assessment of daily activities Assessment of feeding, dressing, washing, toiletting and play must be made when planning therapy (see Chapter 7). However, this overlaps with the assessment of motor developmental channels especially hand function (Chapter 6).

Assessment of equipment includes the selection, the measurements and the assessment of the child in or using the particular piece of equipment.

RECORDS (see 'Grading' above).

Records of assessments and the therapy recommended should be kept despite the difficulties. It is often time-consuming, not accurate, nor reproducible enough from one therapist to the next. (Suggested chart to be used with Grading and accompanying directions. Table 5.3 for method of testing.)

Each child should have a folder with all his assessments and recommendations so that any member of staff can obtain full information. Advice to parents and parent comments should be recorded in this folder so that confusion is avoided and parents given different advice from different staff members.

ASSESSMENT OF TECHNIQUES REQUIRED

As the assessments are made the therapist collects her aims of therapy and daily care and selects techniques from any source to carry these out.

In addition the selected techniques will be assessed during use:

Assessment of techniques chosen *must* take place as one cannot always predict the individual child's response. There must be an *active* response

Table 5.3   Physical Ability Chart (Centre for Spastic Children, 61 Cheyne Walk, London).

Name
Date of birth
Diagnosis

Approximate developmental age level	*Skill*	*Date*	*Rating*
1 week	Prone-head turn to side		
4 weeks	Security on plinth*		
8 weeks	Prone-head raise to just off		
12 weeks	Vertical head control		
16 weeks	Prone-head raise well up		
	Prone—forearm support, head and chest raise		
	Supine—engage hands midline		
	Supine—wriggle 3 feet*		
	Get on to knees and elbows		
	Hold elbows-knees position		
20 weeks	Pull to sit—no head lag		
	Sit, lie down—no head lag		
24 weeks	Prone—come up on extended arms		
	Creep drag lower half*		
	Crawl hands and knees bunny hop*		
	Roll—prone to supine over R.		
	Roll—prone to supine over L.		
	Supine—lift head just off bed		
28 weeks	Supine—lift head well off bed		
	Roll—supine to prone (right)		
	Roll—supine to prone (left)		
	Sit—hands forward for support		
	Stand—held by therapist		
32 weeks	Creep forward—amphibian movement		
36 weeks	Hold hands and knees position		
	Prone—get on to hands and knees		
	Sit—alone on floor		
	Roll—continuous to right		
	Roll—continuous to left		
	Shuffle on buttock*		
	Sit—on ordinary chair		
	Tailor-sitting—no hand support		
	Stand—hold on to furniture		
	Half-kneeling—hands on floor		
	Half-kneeling—upright		
40 weeks	Kneel—sit		

40 weeks	Sitting—go to prone
	Side-sitting lean on one hand
	Prone—get up to side-sitting on floor
	Prone—get up to long-sitting
	Supine—pull up to sitting
	Pull up to stand from chair, hold on
	Pull up to stand from floor, hold on
	Kneel-upright—hold on
44 weeks	Crawl reciprocally
	Stand hold on, lift one foot off floor
48 weeks	Free sitting turn play using hands right
	Free sitting turn play using hands left
	Walk—hold 2 hands
	Walk—mechanical aid (describe)
1 year	Crawl hands and feet
	Walk—one hand held
13 months	Stand alone
1–1½ years	Walk alone
1¼–1½ years	Crawl upstairs
	Get downstairs alone
1¼ years	Kneel upright balance
	Knee-walk
1½ years	Stand up from chair—no support
	Stand up from floor—independently
	Stairs both hands support—ascend
	Stairs both hands upport—descend
	Seat self on knee high chair
	Run
	Stand—pick up object from floor
1¾ years	Climb stairs—hold rail, 2 feet/stair
2 years	Descend stairs—hold rail, 2 feet/stair
	Walk backwards
2½ years	Jump
	Climb stairs alternate feet, hold one hand
	Descend stairs alternate feet, hold one hand
3 years	Climb stairs alternate feet—no hold
	One leg stand 5 secs. right
	One leg stand 5 secs. left
	Hop right
	Hop left
	Stair descent alternately, no hold

---

* Test for independent locomotion, not for training.
Rating system: 1 = no ability;
  2 = partial, laboured, unreliable ability;
  3 = reliable ability, but a grossly abnormal performance;
  4 = reliable ability but with normal or near normal performance.
Note: 'Creeping' is with abdomen on the ground.
  'Crawling' is on hands and knees.

or participation or whenever possible an active initiation on the part of the child with any technique. If not it should be discarded within the first or first few sessions, and another method found. Passive correction of deformities are included but is a small part of the therapy programme. Most passive procedures should in any event *not be totally passive*. They must be assessed to see whether the passive correction manually, with plasters, splintage or bracing makes it possible for *an active* participation of other parts of the child's body or of the particular part of the body being corrected.

APPROACH TO ASSESSMENT

You can obtain the information discussed in the above in a more reliable and more detailed form if you remember the following:

1 Observe the child first in his spontaneous behaviour, at home, school-room and playground. Spontaneous behaviour is quite inadequate and the child does not usually reveal the 'beginning' of a motor ability unless it is specially structured to make him do so in the therapy assessment.

2 In the therapy room, talk to his mother first, while you observe him at play with toys. When the mother accepts you, you will find it easier to assess the child. Also ask the child to bring his favourite toy.

3 There should never be an atmosphere of a 'test' or 'examination' with young children. Much can be obtained during play with the child in his familiar surroundings at home or school.

4 There should be an unhurried atmosphere.

5 Do not undress the child until he is fairly happy about this. Watching him undress will offer excellent assessment of items of posture-balance and hand function.

6 Sequence of the assessment is unimportant. The methodical recording is in sequence but the observations are made according to the child's spontaneous activities and in the order in which he likes to be more formally assessed. This comes with therapy experience. A new therapist tends to start with each channel and fairly methodically collects the items in that channel in the order which they appear. If this is done, do not 'force' the child to keep to this should he become restless.

7 Observations are ongoing so that assessment continues during therapy.

8 You may sometimes begin assessment of main functions, i.e. form of locomotion, ability to sit, stand or walk and rise, and then try some therapy techniques for these functions. Continue assessment alongside therapy techniques in the next sessions.

9 Assessment sessions may take from one to four sessions depending on the child. If therapy is also started the child may reveal more later as he becomes acquainted with his therapist.

10 Many treatment techniques are 'facilitation methods' and so reveal the potential in the child's nervous system whenever this was not obvious at assessment of spontaneous behaviour or even motivating the child to carry out items selected by the therapist.

SUMMARY

1 Assessment is essential for a therapy plan which is relevant to each child.

2 Assessment methods must be selected in *direct* relationship to techniques of treatment. Such a practical approach is outlined in this chapter.

3 Objective valid, reproducible assessments and records still need research.

4 The practical assessment in this chapter includes a developmental functional assessment, examination of deformity (threatening or established), of daily living activities and equipment and can be used for checking progress.

5 Additional assessments of communication, perception and play and social behaviour are also needed.

6 The way in which you approach a child in assessment affects the information obtained. (See also 'Obtaining cooperation of babies and children' on pages 17–19.)

CHAPTER 6

TREATMENT PROCEDURES

MOTOR DEVELOPMENTAL TRAINING

Assessment and techniques

The chapters that follow are presented in relation to the assessment findings of *motor delay*, *abnormal performance* and *reflex reactions*. The assessment findings given are based on much clinical experience. However, there will still be individual problems which cannot all be included in one book.

Developmental levels and techniques

It is important to read chapters 1 and 4 on Developmental Training to understand how to follow and modify normal developmental levels for motor delay and especially motor disorder.

In practice, follow each channel of development for prone, supine, sitting, standing and walking, and hand function. The child may be ahead in one channel and behind in another channel. If some of the postural reactions and voluntary motion cannot be obtained in one channel, attempt them in another. For example:

1 All techniques for head and shoulder control from 0–8 months in normal prone development may also be used with the child's head forward (face towards the ground when necessary), in sitting or standing with table support.

2 All techniques for arm patterns can be carried out in any position, i.e. prone, supine, sitting, standing, kneeling upright.

3 All techniques for pelvic stability may be carried out in prone leading to or alternatively in standing lean hands on a low box. In addition vertical pelvic fixation is trained in the standing positions and upright kneeling. Pelvic stability is trained in supine with 'bridging' technique. Development of sitting does not contribute as much to pelvic control itself, but its contribution of head and trunk control is necessary for pelvic postural fixation on trunk in standing, kneeling and other positions.

4 Supine development may be omitted if head lag is trained through side lying techniques, bringing hands to midline and grasp feet may also be trained in sitting development. Rise from sitting may be omitted if the child can roll over and rise from prone.

5 Development of standing and walking seems to require training in the

standing/walking positions and work in prone/supine contributes little except to correct abnormal joint postures. Sitting development builds up standing in that the head and trunk control developed in sitting will be used in standing.

For most children it is advisable to follow all the developmental channels given. With experience modifications will be obvious with each child and if not the above suggestions may be useful.

Techniques and developmental 'scatter'

It is rare to have techniques from only one developmental stage for *all* the child's motor training. Use the assessment findings on each child and search for his particular problems at the different levels. Remember you will be helping the child:

1 Establish motor abilities at one level with techniques to 'augment' activity.
2 Facilitate motor abilities at the next levels rather than the next level.

Age of child and techniques

In the planning of treatment, there is no special treatment for babies as opposed to children. Select techniques according to developmental level and *not* according to chronological age. Use similar ideas on the treatment of deformity. Commence 'functional training' of feeding, dressing, washing in babies, if they are at the appropriate developmental level.

It is unfortunate that some workers think treatment should be cut down in older children. Postural reactions and other motor controls may only mature much later and unless stimulated will remain dormant. Teachers and other personnel in the older child's life may be shown how to provoke the motor development so that precious school time is not lost from the child's education. The child should not have to miss school in order to travel to physiotherapy departments elsewhere. Some children may have to have specific treatment sessions as special problems arise and before and after orthopaedic surgery. The physiotherapist at the child's school should work out ideas with the teacher to stimulate movement in the classroom, playground or in physical education.

Adjustments to the actual techniques according to the size of child is obvious. However, the same methods may be used for any age. Instructions to babies and children have to be given according to the level of understanding in the baby or child. (See also Obtaining Cooperation in Babies and Children in Chapter 2.)

Onset and techniques

The planning of therapy and selection of techniques is not affected by the onset of the condition at birth, after birth or in later childhood. Response to therapy sometimes seems much quicker if the onset is sudden on a previously normal nervous system. However, ultimately spontaneous recovery and motor development in acquired brain lesions is as unpredictable as in babies born with apparent brain damage. Children with either congenital or acquired lesions warrant stimulation and corrective procedures so that the potential of any of their nervous systems is given every chance to reveal itself. Expectations of better results in children who have 'already known normal movements' may be more of a frustration than a help. It is not so much the memory and experience that matters but the amount of damage *and* the capacity of any particular damaged system to compensate for the abnormalities.

Diagnosis and techniques

The techniques are not devised for particular diagnostic types but for motor problems of delay and abnormal performance. Different diagnostic types may have similar problems and even abnormal performances described may be seen in spastics, athetoids and ataxis as well as other forms of motor delay. This is especially so if abnormal performance is a compensation for delayed balance (postural mechanisms).

Techniques are given for both delay and abnormal performance. Some children may only have motor delay whilst others will have both delay and disorder. Diagnostic features of spasticity, rigidity (hypertonus), involuntary movement, hypotonicity are treated within the treatment suggestions in the motor developmental training as well as in the procedures for the treatment of deformity. (See also Chapter 8.)

Application of techniques

These should be carried out by qualified physiotherapists and occupational therapists and shown to anyone caring for the motor delayed and disabled child. Where techniques require a physiotherapist only, they have been labelled 'physiotherapy suggestions'. Techniques which can be taught to others are labelled 'treatment suggestions and daily care'. Selection of the appropriate technique for each child should be made by therapists and when necessary discussed with doctors and other team members.

Repertoire of techniques in this book cannot possibly include all those available. Firstly, not *all* individual problems could be included together with possible techniques. Secondly, it is difficult to describe techniques without demonstration and only those techniques which could be described have been included. Thirdly, those techniques which have been frequently used have been selected. There are many more.

Lack of response to any technique given in this book indicates the need to try others in this book or in other publications or preferably from clinical colleagues. Check that if the child scarcely responds to any technique, it is not due to:

1   Inaccurate assessment of the child's level of development
2   Inadequate knowledge of the child's non-motor areas of function, i.e. understanding, perception, or other problems which interfere with carrying out movement.
3   Lack of skill of the therapist with the particular technique.

Motor development and child's daily life

Although the techniques below concentrate on the motor problems, they are not isolated from other related areas of function. Wherever possible, motor activities have been interwoven with communication, sensation and perception. Such interactions are particularly obvious in the activities of the child's daily life. Chapter 7 summarises the motor functions trained in this chapter in the contexts of feeding, dressing, playing, toiletting, communication and perceptual experiences.

Although motor abilities in these contexts also train the motor function itself, and makes it even more meaningful to the child, it is often too complex. Motor function needs to be isolated to some degree, to train the deficient motor apparatus. Similarly, perceptual problems or communication (speech and language) problems and special problems of say deafness, blindness should have structured, isolated sessions of training or therapy. Thus therapy has two main aspects.
1   Specialised techniques for specific motor problems to initiate dormant motor activity, intensify correction and training of motor activity.
2   Techniques to integrate motor function with related areas of function in the child's activities of daily living. Integration of movement with perception and cognition.

PRONE DEVELOPMENT

The following main features should be developed:

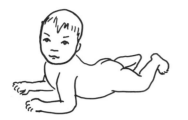

Fig. 6.1 Postural fixation of head and shoulder girdle (on forearms).

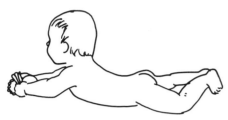

Fig. 6.2 Postural fixation of head and shoulder girdle.

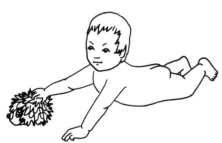

Fig. 6.3 Postural fixation and counterpoising arm reach.

Postural fixation of the head (Figs. 6.1–6.4) when lying prone (0–3 months), on forearms (3 months), on hands and on hands and knees (6 months), during crawling, half-kneeling hand support (9–11 months) or in the 'bear walk' (12 months) in normal developmental levels.

Postural fixation of the shoulder girdle (Figs. 6.2–6.4) when taking weight on forearms (3 months), on hands (6 months), on hands and knees and arms stretched forward along the ground to hold a toy at 5–6 months also include postural fixation. Pivot prone or the 'Landau type' of posture with arms held extended and in the air also provokes postural fixation (8–10 months). Maintenance of half-kneeling lean on hands or upright kneeling lean on hands or grasp a support are other normal developmental motor activities around 9–12 months which stimulate shoulder girdle fixation.

Counterpoising of the head takes place in activities which include head turn and head movements whilst holding the head up against gravity.

Counterpoising the arm movements at about 5 months normal level when in prone lean on one forearm reach with the other or 7 months lean on hand reach with the other (Fig. 6.3). Reach in all directions increases counterpoising ability as well as other features of motor ability.

Postural fixation of the pelvis (Fig. 6.4) on knees with hips at right angles (4 months), on elbows and knees and on hands and knees (4–6 months), on one knee with the other foot flat as in half-kneeling and upright kneeling with support (9–12 months) in normal motor levels.

Counterpoising movement of one leg takes place on knees with upper trunk and arms supported (5–6 months), on hands and knees (6–8 months) together with counterpoising of arm motion in crawling (9–11 months), in bear walk (12 months). Stand lean on hands on low table, carry out leg patterns in each leg also trains counterpoising (12–18 months) in normal developmental levels (see Development of Standing, p. 152).

Rising from prone (Fig. 6.5) head (0–3 months), on to forearms (3 months), on to knees (4 months), on to forearms and knees (5–6 months), on to hands

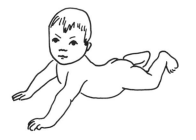 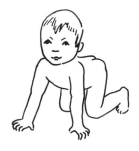

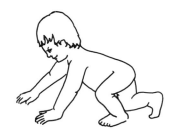

Fig. 6.4 Postural fixation on hands and on hands and knees.

and knees (6–7 months), to half-kneeling hand support (9–12 months), prone to standing without support (12–18 months). Change from and to prone, sitting, squatting, crawling positions (10 months) and other positions with further motor development.

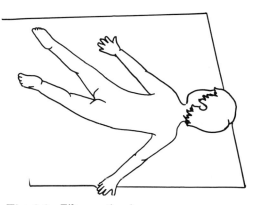

Fig. 6.5 Rising from prone.

Tilt reactions in prone (Fig. 6.6) Reactions seen on tilting the surface on which the child lies at about 6 months; on hands and knees at about 9–12 months.

Saving from falling reactions (Fig. 6.7) in the arms at 5–7 months down-ward-and-forward parachute, and propping. Arms and leg reactions accompany the tilt reactions in prone, especially if the trunk reaction is particularly poor. Other saving reactions are described in the sitting development. Arm saving sideways and forward can also be seen in prone, on hands and knees, if the child is suddenly pushed sideways or forward from a heel-sitting position, or when on hands and knees on a rocking board. Leg reactions also occur on pushing the child over sideways, for-ward, or backward when he is on hands and knees.

0–3 MONTHS NORMAL DEVELOPMENTAL LEVEL

Some common problems

Dislike of prone position This may be due to early breathing difficulties,

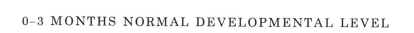

Fig. 6.6 Tilt reaction in prone.

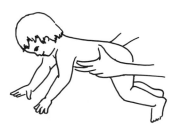

Fig. 6.7 Saving reactions in the arms.

STAGES IN PRONE DEVELOPMENT (Figs. 6.8–6.23)

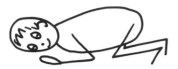

Fig. 6.8   Flexion posture decreases. Head turn (*0–3 months*).

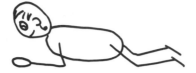

Fig. 6.9   Head raise and hold (*0–3 months*).

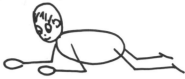

Fig. 6.10   Head raise, weight on forearms (*0–3 months*).

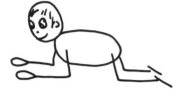

Fig. 6.11   On forearms and/or weight bearing on knees (*3–6 months*).

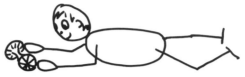

Fig. 6.12   Stretch forward to reach; stretch legs. Lean on one forearm and reach with the other arm (*3–6 months*).

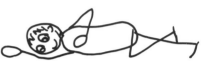

Fig. 6.13   Roll from prone to supine (*3–6 months*).

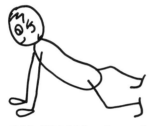

Fig. 6.14   Weight bearing on hands (*6–9 months*).

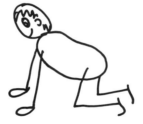

Fig. 6.15   Weight bearing on hands and knees (*6–9 months*).

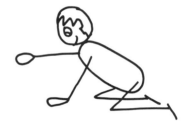

Fig. 6.16   Lean on one hand reach with the other (*7 months*).

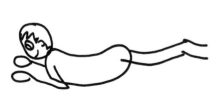

Fig. 6.17   Extend head, shoulders, hips—pivot prone position (*8 months*).

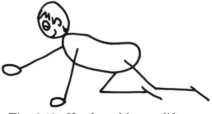

Fig. 6.18   Hands and knees, lift arm, leg or both (*8 months*).

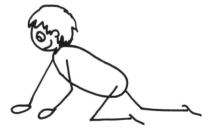

Fig. 6.19   Crawling (*9 months*).

Changing positions constantly—prone to sit: to crawl: to squat: to supine

Fig. 6.20

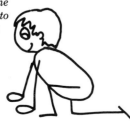

Fig. 6.21   Half-kneeling lean on hands (*11 months*).

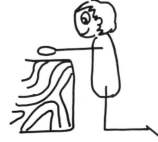

Fig. 6.22   Kneeling supported (*11 months*).

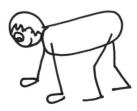

Fig. 6.23   Bear-walk (elephant walk) on hands and feet (*12 months*).

inability to turn the head and free the nose, inability to lift the head up, excessive flexion creating discomfort in prone or even lack of opportunity given to lie on his stomach. Later a dislike of prone may be due to the child's inability to use his hands in prone.

Delayed development of head control, rising up on forearms, taking weight on forearms.

Abnormal performance (Fig. 6.24), e.g. asymmetrical head raise, rising on one forearm only, asymmetrical stabilisation on elbows, excessive flexion of either of the arms (often caught under the child's body), the trunk or legs, or all of them. There may be more flexion-adduction in one leg than the other as the hips lift off the surface into flexion. One leg may flex and abduct into a forward creeping pattern with hips flexed off the surface or flat. This asymmetry of flexion is often greater in spastic diplegia than in quadriplegia. Athetoid quadriplegia and floppy babies tend to flex and abduct both legs outwards into the 'frog position'. Hemiplegic children begin to creep and flex the good side whilst the hemiplegic side goes into extension—internal rotation. This is seen especially when the child raises his head and turns to the good side. Independent head raising in the other cerebral palsied children is usually associated with flexion in the arms but extension of the back and especially of the legs into adduction-internal

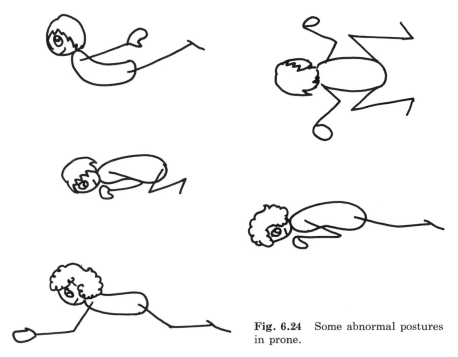

Fig. 6.24 Some abnormal postures in prone.

rotation. In normal babies the leg extension (especially at the next developmental level) is associated with abduction and external rotation.

Reflex reactions in prone   Reaction to prone: arm flexor reaction: Galant's response, neck righting not beginning to diminish. Appearance of head righting may be delayed.

Treatment suggestions and daily care

Acceptance of prone position   Accustom the child to prone by placing him slowly on his stomach and on soft surfaces, such as sponge rubber, inflatable mattress, in warm water, over large rubber beach ball, over your lap (adding a cushion if your knees are bony!). Gently bring his bent arms away from his chest and place them over an edge or curved surface, rock and sway a baby held in prone suspension. The child's face should be over the edge of the surface with the nose free. Training should be given to help him turn his head to the side, if he cannot do this (see below).

The child may also be suspended in a blanket or hammock and gently rolled from sidelying into pronelying and back until he accepts that last roll into prone lying. His nose should be over the edge of the blanket as he rolls over.

Note   Some children continue to strongly refuse to go prone and should not be forced to do so. Some of these are like normal children who are 'rollers' or 'bottom shufflers' and a few others who do not use prone development in their motor behaviour (Robson) [23].

Head control   Train these aspects of head control:
—raising the head (righting)
—holding the head steady (postural fixation)
—turning the head from side to side (counterpoising and movement)
1   Place the child in prone across a sponge rubber roll, a beach ball, a wedge, pile of pillows or across your lap. Then elevate his arms and gently stretch them symmetrically across the surface or over the edge of the surface. Stiff arms may first have to be grasped near the shoulder joints and turned outwards as they are extended forwards over the edge of the apparatus or on the ball. The child's legs may be abnormally bent or stiffly extended, turned in and held together, before or only during head raising. In such cases turn them out and keep his legs apart *while* he is obtaining head control (Fig. 6.25).

Rock the child forward and backwards over the edge of the roll/ball or inflatable mattress. Rhythmically tap under the child's chin to give momen-

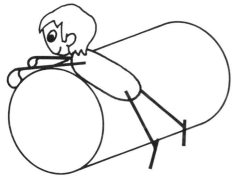

Fig. 6.25

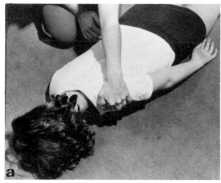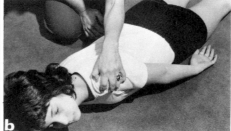

Fig. 6.26

tum to lift the head. Tapping the child's forehead also helps if he does not like having his face touched. Hold the child's shoulders on both sides symmetrically.

2   Bring his shoulders back and inwards towards his spine—this provokes him to head raise. If the child persists in abnormal turning of his head to one side, then extend the shoulder girdle on the opposite side to provoke head turn and raise to that side (Fig. 6.26).

3   With the child's head over the edge present him with interesting visual and auditory stimuli, slightly above him and also in front of him. Provoke head raise and hold in various positions (Fig. 6.27). If the child raises his head slightly to one side, place stimuli on the other side. Stimulate the child to look up at interesting objects such as mobiles, Christmas decorations, mirrors, moving toys on springs or mechanically controlled, sounds from musical boxes, squeaky toys and mother's voice. At first use stimuli in the centre and progress to having them at each side of the child and move them slowly from centre to the side and from side to side. These stimuli obtain head control and eye fixation and tracking so that training of head control associates with vision and also hearing (pages 17, 36).

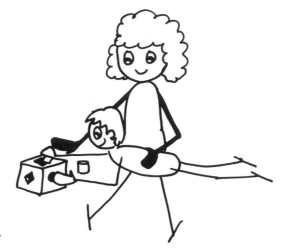

Fig. 6.27

4 Place wedge on a table or platform so that the child can see the adult's face when he looks up. The adult obtains eye-to-eye contact by sitting in the centre and opposite the child, and sings or speaks to him.

5 Keep wedge on the floor or in a sandpit or in front of a trough of water where other children are playing.

6 Place child in prone on an inflatable mattress, large ball, water bed or trampoline and gently bounce him to provoke head raise.

7 Swing baby in prone over adult's arms or large child on a horizontal tyre suspended from a tree. Help child to go down a slide while lying prone on a cushion. Place child on a wedge on wheels or on a trolly with a roll of towels between his body and upper arms.

8 Weight bearing on forearms will also help the child's head control (Fig. 6.28).

Use all visual and auditory stimuli in these positions as above. Check that the child's forearms are well away from the body, with elbows at right angles to body and, if possible, hands open. If the child's elbows still pull back against his body, place a roll of towels between his body and his upper arms. Check good position of head trunk and legs (head and trunk centre, in alignment, legs apart, straight, turned out from hips).

Fig. 6.28 Head control and weight bearing on forearms (on elbows). Prone, on forearms over low wedge, roll cushions. Keep legs apart and turned out in those cases where legs press together and/or twist inwards. Use a pommel, toy, small wedge or cushion for legs.

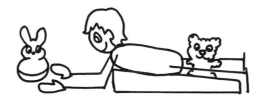

Equal weight on forearms   Weight bearing is often better on one side.

1   Encourage the use of the more affected side by gently pushing the child's weight over it, whilst he is preoccupied with play. Also place toys in such a way that he leans on to the unstable side and uses his other arm to play. An older child should be told, but not nagged, to do this as well. Give the child a toy to use with one arm while you gently push his weight over and hold him on to the weaker weight-bearing side. As soon as possible remove your support and do not hold him during play. Do this also during feeding, washing and other activities in sitting (p. 194).

2   When the child is in prone lying over a roll, pillows or wedge, press down firmly through his head in line with his neck, or down through the top of his shoulders increasing his weight bearing on to his elbows (see Figures 6.97, 6.98).

3   Hold baby with his full weight through his elbows or on one elbow. Slightly shift his weight, first on to one elbow and then on to the other elbow. An older child can do this if you hold his legs up in the air while he takes weight on to his forearms. Hold a spastic's legs apart, turned outward and with straight hips and knees.

Note   Always try removing any supports given by your hands or equipment to check whether the child can lift his head or take weight on forearms on his own momentarily and with practice reliably.

Physiotherapy suggestions

Abnormal postures   Excessive flexion and other abnormal postures are corrected by the stimulation of head raise symmetrically, head turn to non-preferred side, weight bearing on forearms at right-angles to chest, stretching child out symmetrically over rolls, wedges, mother's lap and active extension movements and the active creeping patterns. General corrective positioning and splintage may be needed (pp. 81, 83, 91).

1   *Facilitate symmetrical head raising* by either holding both the child's shoulders in rotation-extension or both arms elevated, abducted-external rotation behind the plane of his head or by asking him to push his elevated arms back against your hands pressing against his upper arms and straight elbows, or by use of the creeping arm pattern carried out in the plane behind the child's head.

2   *Facilitate head raise and turn* as in Fig. 6.26 or by lifting the elevated arm on one side back and behind the child's head provokes the creeping pattern, Fig. 6.29a, in one leg.

3   *Facilitate rising on to one elbow* as in supine development from side-lying (Fig. 6.60) or within creeping pattern.

Creeping patterns   It is difficult to describe these patterns without demonstration. Some aspects will be described as these techniques are particularly helpful.

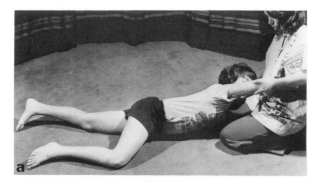

Fig. 6.29

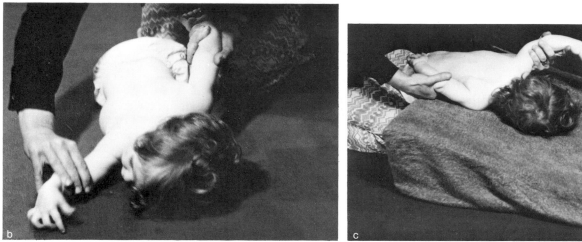

The 'face arm' is elevated into shoulder abduction-external rotation (Fig. 6.29b). The 'occiput arm' is brought down into shoulder extension-adduction internal rotation (Fig. 6.29c). The child may lie flat on the surface or over the edge of a roll, small pillow or wedge.

1 Assisted active changing of the arms so that the opposite arm is elevated whilst the 'face arm' moves down facilitates head raise and turn, back extension and leg creeping movements.

2 Use of stretch-rotation and appropriate resistance activates the creeping movements.

3 The child may continue active creeping on his own and so acquire one form of locomotion beginning at this level of development.

4 If the elevated 'face arm' is held stationary by your hand or a firm padded object, you can concentrate on facilitating the creeping forward action of the 'occiput arm' against your manual or just thumb resistance. If the child understands, ask him to pull his arm forward and above his head. An automatic rising reaction on to the forearm of the 'face arm' occurs. In some babies and severely affected older children, the stretch of the 'occiput arm' especially with extension-rotation of the shoulder girdle on that side, provokes the same automatic rise on to the forearm of the 'face arm'. As the child rises, he also raises and turns his head.

5 Facilitation of leg creeping involves single leg flexion-abduction-external rotation, preferably with pelvic rotation backward. The other leg is held in extension-adduction-*external* rotation. Legs should be held at the thigh and knee using stretch-rotation and resistance according to the child's reaction. (See also Fig. 29a.)

6 Like arm creeping, the facilitation of the leg motion counteracts abnormal postures of the legs, trunk flexion and arm flexion against chest (arm flexor reaction; reaction to prone).

Active leg creeping may facilitate active automatic arm creeping actions. For example, hold one of the child's legs at the thigh and knee and stretch it into extension-adduction external rotation. A quick stretch into into this pattern provokes a 'recoil' towards flexion-abduction-external rotation which is the forward creeping motion of the leg. If the child understands, ask him to bend his hip and knee up and out against your hand. Offer him enough resistance to augment his movement.

As the leg creeps forward and especially if it is guided into full external rotation with pelvic rotation backwards, there is an automatic arm creeping forward, usually on the same side or on the contralateral (opposite) side. This creeping technique is useful for activation of more affected arms or arm as in hemiplegic babies or mentally subnormal severely affected children.

7 Rising reactions may be provoked if the flexion-abduction-externally rotated leg is held fixed manually or by a padded box. The other leg is provoked into flexion-abduction-external rotation as above. The effect may be rising on to the forearms, the hands or the knee on the fixed or stationary side. Rising on to knees is more likely in children in the developmental level of 4–6 months. (See Fig. 6.33 at the next level of development.)

There are many possibilities for rising reactions and other stabilising and movement reactions with Vojta's creeping techniques and my own modifications. However, they have to be demonstrated and supervision given by specialised phasiotherapists.

Facilitate rising on to both forearms or later hands at the same time. Hold the child's head by spanning his occiput between his ears. Ask him to raise his head up against your manual pressure. This pressure and sometimes manual resistance facilitates rising on to his forearms or hands.

Augment head holding, and forearm support by resistance to head hold, as well as head raise. Encourage child to pull his chin inwards getting 'a long neck'. Also give manual resistance to front, side, back of shoulders, as child is told to '*stay there*' or '*don't let me push you down*' or simply '*hold it*'.

Note Use of resistance is recommended for athetoids and ataxics and weak developmentally disabled children. In spastics, resistance should be controlled so that there is no abnormal overflow such as extensor spasms or flexor spasms.

4–6 MONTHS NORMAL DEVELOPMENTAL LEVEL

Common problems

Delay in acquisition of rising on knees, rising on to hands with straight elbows, weight bearing on knees, knees and forearms and on one forearm, reaching for objects, inability to lie prone with both or one of the arms stretched and reaching overhead, unable to roll over to supine, or unable to creep on abdomen, on elbows or with various creeping movements of both arms and legs.

Abnormal performance   Asymmetric, abnormal positions of limbs, clenching hands during the activities, beginning 'mermaid crawl' (see 6–9 months' level).

Abnormal rising patterns in prone include child pulling his knees up under his abdomen on his forearm support, then pushing up on to his hands; child rising on to his knees only with head and trunk flexed over bent arms; arms may not be used at all or he pushes up on semiflexed arms with clenched or open hands; child rising on to hands first and using his hands to push himself backwards into heel sitting.

All these patterns are only abnormal if it indicates lack of weight bearing on hands with straight elbows, or on knees with hip fixation at 90°. Otherwise they need not be corrected by the therapist.

Reflex reactions may persist from earlier level.

Treatment suggestions and daily care

Rising on to knees   Encourage the child's rising on to knees instead of your lifting the child each time. Place one leg in creeping position and hold firmly or fix the leg against a heavy box, tip the child's *opposite* hip and pelvis up and back with a slight touch and wait for active automatic rise on to knees, first on to the one that is fixed. The other leg creeps forward on to its knee. Carry this out without giving the child a 'tip-up' at his hip, *if he can manage alone* as in Fig. 6.30.

Weight bearing on knees, on forearms and knees (4–6 months), on hands and knees, on hands, abdomen, on the ground or wedge (6–9 months)

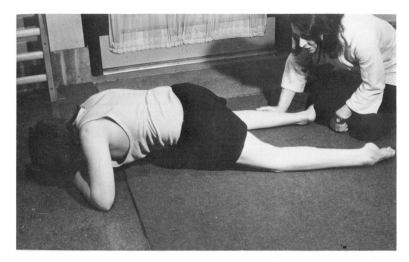

Fig. 6.30

(Fig. 6.31). Place the child on his knees, knees and forearms or hands and knees or on his hands with straight elbows with abdomen on the ground or support, according to his level of development.

1   If there is tightness of hips and knee flexors, use on hands support with abdomen and legs straight.

2   Use your lap, wedges, rolls, pillows, suspension in a blanket, sponge rubber shapes or big soft toys for support until the child can balance alone.

3   Use visual stimuli, toys, balls, sand and water play in these positions.

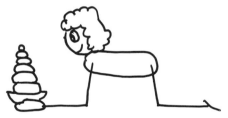

Fig. 6.31

4   Have hips at right angles when he takes weight on his knees. Increase the activities with the arms during weight bearing on knees. Active use of the hands provokes greater weight bearing on knees for stability.

5   Press down on the child's lower back and buttocks to increase his weight bearing on his knees, and if his knees slide during his play with his hands, or 'shoot out into extension'.

6   Use elbow splints to help weight bearing on hands with straight elbows. Magazines may initially hold the elbows straight so that shoulders develop stability during these weight bearing activities.

7   Open the child's hands by pressing his weight through the heels of his hands; by gently bringing the thumbs out from their bases and not from their tips and by joint compression through the length of the arm.

Unstable weight bearing through the arms (Fig. 6.32)   Joint compression through the arm to provoke stability (co-contraction). Press through the top of the child's shoulder and/or through the straight elbow. Arm must be in straight alignment with the line of pressure through shoulder or elbow. Keep weight through heel of his hand to avoid finger flexion. Arms may also be placed on a surface below the child so that the weight of his body adds to the joint compression, e.g. on a stool below the plinth on which

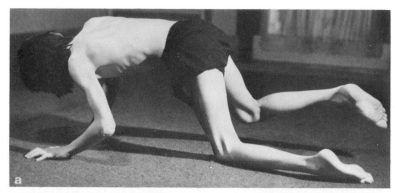

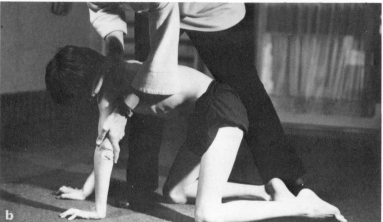

Fig. 6.32

he lies upon. Child 'Walks on hands' with his elbow splints, for similar effects.

1 Weight bearing on one forearm, reach with the other. Weight bear and shift from forearm to forearm. Encourage reach with one arm on floor, then above his head and in different positions. Hold and bring object to mouth and similar single arm movements carried out whilst weight bearing on the other arm.

2 With the child bearing weight on both forearms give him toys in each hand to grasp and play with. Let him grasp the ends of a bicycle pump, concertina, plastic bottle, transparent cylinder with coloured water or marbles inside, grasp two balls or blocks to bang together or push a ball from hand to hand. Toys should move or make a noise if touched, patted, pressed or grasped. Remove the wedge and hold the child on one of his forearms while he actively uses the other arm in play. Whenever possible remove adult support altogether (see Development of Hand Function).

3 Child in prone lying on forearms on thick soft sponge, inflatable mattress, water bed, trampoline, press the surface down on each side so that the child tips on to his elbow. Do this to a song or rhythm.

4 Child may weight shift from one forearm to the other forearm in order to creep along the floor. As the child creeps on his abdomen with weight shift on the forearms it is best if the legs are held up, turned out and apart in cases where the legs stiffen into abnormal positions with thighs pressed together or turned in during this activity of creeping or 'walking on the elbows' or 'wheelbarrow on forearms'. You can also place the child on a low platform or low wedge on wheels with the legs held in abduction with abduction pants or a pommel. The child should be shown how to use his 'elbow walking' *backwards*. If he is on a bed and wishes to get off he could then move himself backwards so that his legs come off the edge of the bed, his feet take the weight and he can stand up leaning on elbows.

Note   Do *not* use this activity in those cases where there is a tendency to tight elbow flexion and shoulder hunching but rather practise weight bearing on one elbow stretching out for toys with the other arm and also stretching both arms well forward to toy or to push a big ball away.

Arms stretched overhead and forward: arm saving reactions in prone: propping reactions
1   Encourage the child to reach forward and overhead for toys, to push away a ball, balloon or toy on wheels. Older children can 'walk' their hands up a wall or wall bars as far as possible (Fig. 8.1). Use a small bolster or wedge to help him stretch his arms out *and* up towards toys on a box or suspended above him.
2   Place the child over a beach ball or large roll with his arms over the top. Tip the ball forward and encourage him to reach for the ground to save himself from falling. Encourage him to prop himself on his hands by placing his hands on the ground, to 'stand on his hands' whilst you hold his body safely on the ball. You can hold a young child and tip him upside down near a surface, e.g. a table, and encourage him to put his arms out to save himself and then to take weight on them (Fig. 6.47).
3   Place the child on his abdomen on a large cushion with his arms stretched forward, and help him to go down a slide 'head first'. Also tip a horizontal stationary cushion downwards to provoke arm saving reaction.

Note   The therapist must check whether positions of arms and legs are correct during all the activities above, e.g.:
—shoulders and hips at right angles in weight bearing positions
—knees pointed outwards
—hips and knees straight, apart, and if possible turned outwards
—shoulders and arms turned out rather than inward
—hands open and palms down if weight bearing
It is important to recognise that *all the training* of weight bearing on elbows, one elbow, hands may be done in *sitting or standing* leaning forward down on to a low table or box. This reinforces the prone development *or* if prone is occasionally not indicated for a particular child, these activities can and should be trained in these other positions.

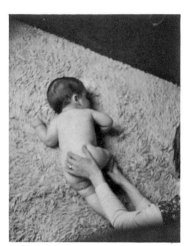

Fig. 6.33

Rolling from prone to supine   See Rolling Techniques.

Physiotherapy suggestions

Facilitate rising for assumption of four-point position (forearms and knee position)

1   Fix one of the child's legs in creeping position with a box or manually (Fig. 6.33). Press down through his buttocks. You may hold his other leg above or below the knee and stretch it into extension—adduction—external rotation provoking a creeping movement forward. If the child understands he should be instructed to 'bend' his hip and knee. If this movement is fully resisted by the therapist no movement occurs but instead the child will right or rise up on his other knee, or on to his arms.

Note the automatic creeping forward of this baby's right arm.

2   Hold the child under his upper arms. Rotate his arms and his trunk to one side to facilitate creeping forward of one leg. Rotate him to the other side so that he rises up onto both knees.

3   When the child is actively able to commence or even complete rising up onto knees and forearms, but is weak, then resistance is used to reinforce his efforts. Apply manual resistance at the pelvis in a diagonal direction (Fig. 6.34).

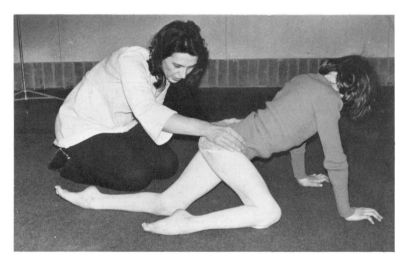

Fig. 6.34

See roll-and-rise (Fig. 6.67).

Facilitate rising on to hands by using the same techniques as rising on to elbows at 0–3 months level above, but this time expecting child to rise all the way on to hands.

Augment holding on hands and knees

1   The child attempts to maintain this position as the therapist slowly pushes him:

—laterally at each hip or each shoulder
—anteroposteriorly at hip or shoulders
—at opposite shoulder and hip
—at shoulder and hip on the same side
2 Resistance to head movements and to shoulders 'stay there' (see on forearms, page 79). Similarly use resistance for hips when child is on knees with chest and arms supported by roll or stool.

6–9 MONTHS NORMAL DEVELOPMENTAL LEVEL

Common problems

Delay in weight bearing on hands and knees, in lifting one or two limbs, weight bearing on one hand and reaching for objects, crawling on hands or on knees, pivot position and absence of rising from prone to hands and knees.

Abnormal performance of motor abilities, over-flexed hips, knees or feet, internally rotated legs or arms, lack of reciprocation in crawling, 'bunny hopping' both knees forward in heel sitting, asymmetrical weight bearing. Prone 'mermaid crawl' or 'commando crawl' by pulling forward on his flexed arms with his legs stiffly extended, adducted and internally rotated. The hands may clench with each 'pull' forward and often the legs adduct strongly with this pull.

Absence of reflex reactions expected at 6–9 months level in prone, absence of Landau, saving reactions in arms, tilting reactions in prone. Persistence of any early reactions, see 0–3 months level.

Lack of postural fixation of the pelvis and hips creates creeping on the abdomen and masks the child's ability to take weight on hands at 6 months level of development.

Flexion or lack of postural fixation of head, shoulder girdle and hips in extension or flexion positions may be treated with techniques above or with pivot prone (Fig. 6.35). Pivot prone or Landau position provoked by head raise:
—this can also be carried out on a large ball, roll
—also elevate-abduct-externally rotate arms behind plane of head
—abduct-extend and externally rotate legs in this child when she is on a roll
—older children may abduct-externally rotate shoulders in postural fixation by pulling against weights over pulleys opposite them. Abdomen on low stool which supports the child at the chest and abdomen but allows extension in head and limbs is used.

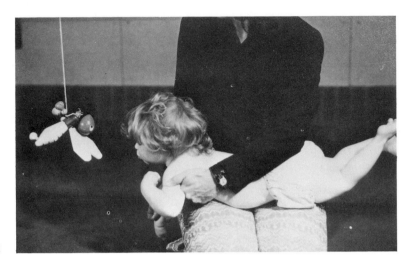

Fig. 6.35

Note The extension in pivot prone is not enough for standing. Postural fixation of the head, trunk and hips in the vertical must be trained (see Development of Standing, p. 135).

Treatment suggestions and daily care
See Figs. 6.31 and 6.32 and add the following.

Weight bearing on one hand, reach for a toy and on hands and knees lift one arm or leg or both Place the child on hands or on hands and knees over rolls or your arm and when possible let him balance on his own:
1   Lift individual limbs whilst he maintains balance to a song or counts.
2   While child takes weight on his hands or hands and knees, encourage him to stroke different textures on the ground, e.g. carpets, linoleum, cool and warm surfaces, scratchy and smooth surfaces.
3   While balancing on hands and knees he might scrub the floor or soap the linoleum, reach for a dangling toy, roll balls, move small toys on wheels, dig into the sandpit with one hand or a spade, on the grass he could pick flowers, handfuls of grass and so on.

Crawling This can be trained with the child:
1   Suspended in a blanket. Hold each end of the blanket and tip the child in it so that his weight is taken more on one side releasing the other side for a 'step' forward.
2   On a crawler. Hold the child's knees and point them outwards. Move one knee in front of the other. Tip the child onto the weight bearing knee as you guide the moving knee.

Note It is important to avoid the use of crawlers and the training of crawling in children who have tight hip and knee flexors. In these cases use a wedge on wheels or platform on wheels with towels rolled under the child's chest so that his elbows are straight and his arms reach for the floor. The child crawls on his hands whilst his legs are held extended on the platform. See also 'wheelbarrow' on forearms (page 83) and do the same but as 'wheelbarrow on hands'. In cases of severe knee and elbow flexion, splintage of these joints should be used as the child gets about on his platform on wheels.

Rolling Encourage rolling on grass down a slight incline, on sponge rubber, on an inflatable mattress or down a mound (see Rolling Techniques, and Roll-and rise, page 103).

Physiotherapy suggestions
Child maintains balance on:

Hands and knees and carries out arm or leg patterns to achieve counter-poising (Fig. 6.36).

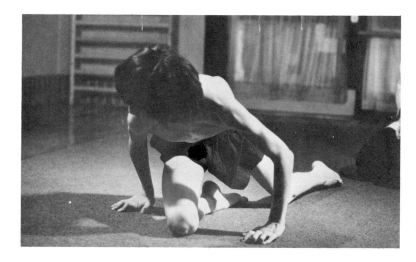

Fig. 6.36 Instability of pelvic and shoulder girdles and counter poising.

Leg pattern Ask the child to bend one knee up to the ceiling; manually resist his knee flexion forward and outward. Then reverse to hip and knee extension with adduction and external rotation (Fig. 6.37–6.39). Resistance given to leg pattern will also increase stabilisation at the shoulder girdle and opposite hip.

Arm pattern Use creeping pattern of child's arm from extension-adduction-internal rotation behind his back, facilitated to elevation-abduction-

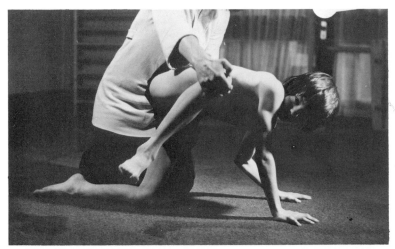

Fig. 6.37

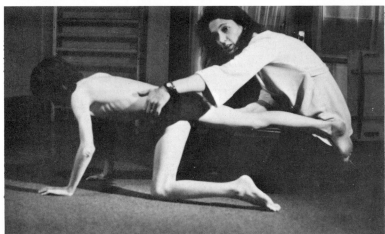

Fig. 6.38

Fig. 6.39 Positions of therapist's hands. Child's leg flexion against hand on thigh or pull against hand on tibia. Leg extension against hand on tibia.

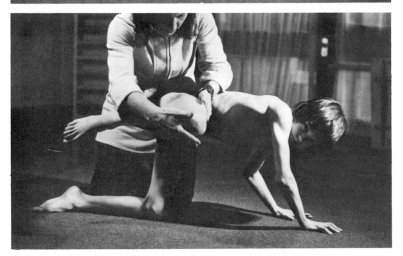

external rotation as described at the earlier levels (Fig. 6.29). Other arm patterns are arm flexion adduction across chest, change to abduction-extension-external rotation with trunk rotation backwards. As the child moves his one arm against resistance, he increases weight bearing or stabilisation on the other three points. If he is on his hands only, abdomen on the floor, shoulder stabilisation and counterpoising is stimulated, as follows: he balances on the one hand as single arm pattern of movement is carried out actively or against correctly given resistance.

1 Continue pivotting in flexed children as above (Fig. 6.35).
2 Continue rising on to hands *and* knees as above or roll-and-rise (p. 102).
3 Child crawls against resistance given to his knees. Grasp his knees and guide them outward as you resist each step forward (Fig. 6.40).
4 Augment holding on hands and knees (as above), especially the hips in 'bunny hoppers'. Suggestions to discourage 'bunny hopping' are given below.

Items **3** and **4** overlap into next stage of development.

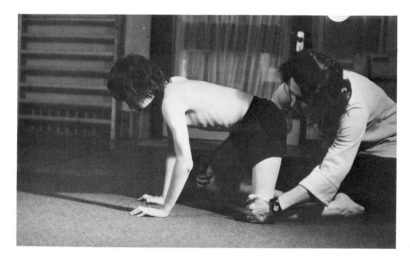

Fig. 6.40

9–12 MONTHS NORMAL DEVELOPMENTAL LEVEL

Common problems

Delay in easy reciprocal crawling, maintaining half-kneeling position hands on ground, on hands and feet and other more advanced postures. Absence of rising from hands and knees to standing holding a support and inability to change from prone to sitting, prone to squatting, prone to supported half-kneeling; grasping support or hands on floor and other changes of posture.

Abnormal performance Spastic adduction-internal rotation of hips in crawling, in half-kneeling and weight bearing on hands and feet. If the child can 'bear walk' on hands and feet, he has his heels off the ground and/ or excessive flexion of the knees with hips internally rotated and adducted.

Absence of reflex reactions expected at 9–12 months in prone, Landau, saving reaction in arms fully developed. Persistence of any earlier reflex reactions, see previous levels.

Treatment suggestions and daily care

Half-kneeling Sit the child on the side of your lap when you sit on the ground. Bring his outside knee on to the floor, he is then kneeling on one knee, hold the other knee forward and outward. Remove your lap and place his hands on the floor for support. Encourage him to play in this position by moving a car or rolling a ball under the 'bridge' of his knee, round his foot, or spend time in tying his boot laces, count his toes, paint his toe nails and so on. Later, he should grasp horizontal bars, at various levels, place his hands flat on the wall, low tables or your flat hands. Half-kneeling position should be maintained with the front knee pointing outward. Hold his knee out with his foot pointing out and placed out to the side. This is often difficult. Ask the child to press his front knee outwards against your hand and also maintain balance. Augment his balance by offering manual resistance to his hips at the side, shoulder girdle at the side and shoulder and hip girdles at the same time.

Whilst on hands in half-kneeling and also in upright half-kneeling, grasp a support. Manual resistance may also be used. In addition head lift against resistance applied between his ears across the lower occiput helps to augment the stabilisation.

Rising from prone to standing Once the half-kneeling position is assumed it should continue as a transitional position on the way to standing up. Assumption of half-kneeling takes place using the exercise in Figs. 6.37– 6.39. In Fig. 6.41 the therapist is helping the child place his foot flat on the ground. Fig. 6.42 shows how to hold the knee and foot steady as the child rises. Another method is to hold the child's body under his chest whilst he controls his limbs, or for the child to grasp supports from the hands and knees position and pull himself up to standing via the half-kneeling position. You may also ask the child to rise against your hand pressing his lower back and pelvis as in Fig. 6.42.

Note The application of manual resistance must be done by physiotherapists as careful control of any abnormal overflow, the correct amount of resistance and technique of application is important.

See also other patterns of rising from prone in the chart on page 165.

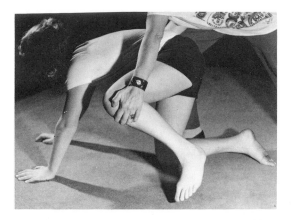

Fig. 6.41

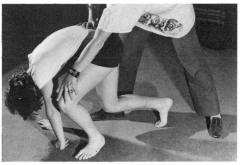

Fig. 6.42

Weight taken on hands and feet and 'bear walk' The child may place his hands on a low stool if he cannot easily reach the ground. Stabilisation together with gentle passive stretching of tight hamstrings is carried out in this position. In addition the counterpoising exercises in Figs. 6.37–6.39 should be done in this position and are illustrated in the Development of Standing at the 9–12 month developmental level (p. 155).

Stepping on hands and feet can be carried out using a stool on wheels, a low chair on sliding skis, with a sledge or stable wooden toy on wheels. Hold the child's thighs and knees straight and turned outward if there is any abnormal flexion-adduction-internal rotation. Give manual resistance to the stepping leg whilst holding the standing knee straight, to stretch tight hamstrings or increase the action of the fixators of the hip. Wearing knee gaiters for the 'bear walk' or for slow upright stepping, prevents the use of knee flexion *and* also activates the stabilisers (postural fixators) of the pelvic girdle. Joint compression through hips or knees of the standing leg also helps this stability.

Many normal children do not 'bear walk' but the cerebral palsied and motor delayed child needs this motor activity for stabilisation of shoulder girdle (lean on hands) and pelvic girdle, stretching of tight hamstrings, stretching of tight heel cords (heels kept flat on the ground) as well as the counterpoising of each limb as a step is taken.

Hyperextended knees may be treated in the bear walk (see Fig. 6.164).

Increasing stability of the hips is associated with a decrease of hyperextension of the knees which may be a compensation for lack of fixation at the hips.

Tilt reactions and saving reactions in limbs on hands and knees may be stimulated on a rocker board, inflatable mattress or thick soft sponge rubber (Fig. 6.43).

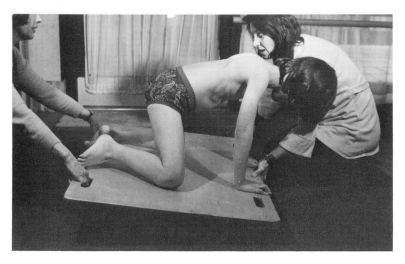

Fig. 6.43

Changes of posture from prone kneeling (on hands and knees) to sitting and back again, to prone lying and back again, to half-kneeling and back again and many other changes as in the righting reactions, should be trained at this level of development. See the development of sitting at this level. These activities overlap into all the other channels.

Problem of 'bunny hopping'   Reciprocal crawling rather than the continual 'bunny hopping' of both knees forward should be present by this level. Unstable pelvis, excessive spasticity in hip and knee flexors and also habit prolongs bunny hopping and aggravates these problems, as well as adding deformities of the feet. Discourage bunny hopping by offering other means of locomotion such as the prone board on casters for prone lying with hips and knees straight, a tricycle, pedal car, crawler and preferably walkers, with knees in gaiters, if necessary. Training children to 'bottom shuffle' is also a good alternative and easily accepted by many children. The child sits with feet in front on the ground. He leans on his hands at his sides, presses his feet flat on the ground and stretches out his knees and moves along the ground, backwards, or forwards.

Encourage crawling on all surfaces, sand, grass, carpets, tiles, as well as using crawling on to a large step made with mattresses, wood or concrete, and climb in and out of boxes, cubby holes, through tunnels and under tables etc.

Discourage crawling in children with tight hip and knee flexors and equinus feet.

Training upright kneeling This is discussed here as the child rises from prone positions to this position. Kneeling upright holding on to a support is expected at about 9–12 months whilst kneeling alone only at about 15 months in normal child development (Gesell).

Do not use this position in children who persist with hip flexion, lordosis or hip-knee-dorsiflexion in this position. Control this by pressure against the extended hip and keeping the knees at right angles. The back is held straight by the child leaning his trunk against a sofa or holding the arms forward in flexion, elbows straight and lean or grasp a support. However all this may not really control every child's deformities.

Use upright kneeling if the abnormalities can be controlled (usually in athetoids and ataxics and motor delayed children) to develop vertical pelvic fixation and postural fixation of trunk on pelvis before standing supported is possible. Usually standing supported *is* possible if well controlled and is preferable. However, in children with deformities of the feet, plantigrade feet are not available for the standing position. Upright kneeling achievement in such a child confirms the need for surgery or plasters for the feet which are then preventing standing. Naturally knee flexors must also be checked for deformity.

Upright kneeling balance in kneel standing, knee walking sideways and forwards and backwards and kneeling on a rocker board may be useful in some children if for any reason these activities cannot be carried out in standing.

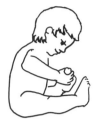

Fig. 6.44 Postural fixation and counterpoising of the limbs.

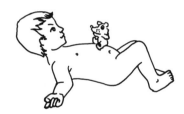

Fig. 6.45   Rising from supine.

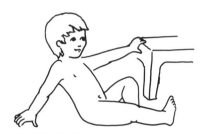

Fig. 6.46   Postural fixation of the head.

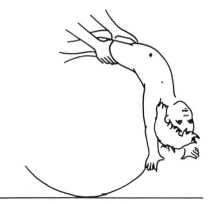

Fig. 6.47   Arms saving (parachute) reaction from supine.

SUPINE DEVELOPMENT

The following main features should be developed:

Postural fixation of the shoulder girdle as the child holds the arm up in the air for reach, reach and grasp and other hand function and hand–eye coordination (page 185), beginning about 4 months normally when the hands are held in midline in, say, 'hand regard', at 5 months during reach for an object.

Postural fixation of the pelvis as the child holds a leg up in the air, say, at 7 months in order to grasp his foot with his hand; at 5 months when a child 'bridges' his hips off the surface *without* using back extensor spasm to do so.

Counterpoising the limbs in the air (Fig. 6.44)   Children who cannot do this tip over when they are on their backs in water. Thus, holding a limb up in the air with absence of a hard surface increases a demand on the musculature needed for counterpoising, and reveals its inadequacy. Developmental level may be about 5–7 months when normal children hold their limbs steady in the air.

Rising reactions (Fig. 6.45)   These are probably the most important reactions or activities to be trained in supine development. Many abnormal postures and abnormal reactions are particularly obvious in supine. Training the child to get out of supine includes counteracting most of these reactions. This training seems to be preferable than spending time correcting the child's position in supine. Supine, *head rising* (righting) and the *overcoming of head lag* prepares and trains rising out of supine. Various *rolling-and-rising* reactions e.g. roll and rise onto hands and knees, roll to prone and rise; roll half-way to side-lying or side-sitting; roll half-way and grasp a support and pull to sitting or standing, should be trained. If these are impossible, other patterns must be found as, say, in the athetoid child in Fig. 6.71. Rising is important as supine is a position of particular helplessness.

Postural fixation of the head (Fig. 6.46) is not head raising and requires special training. Head control is raising *and* holding of the head as well a head turning. Head holding is expected at 4–6 months normally, either, in supine on the surface with head held off the surface, or, if the baby is held suspended horizontally in supine and he holds his head alone in this position in midline.

Note   Normal asymmetries, abnormal asymmetries and other aspects are discussed below. Pivoting on the back by movements of the arms and legs so that the child can move in circles may also be required in some children. *Tilt reactions* and *saving reactions* (Fig. 6.47) are less important in supine than in sitting and standing.

STAGES IN SUPINE DEVELOPMENT (Figs. 6.48–6.57)

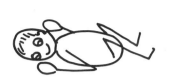

Fig. 6.48 Flexion: asymmetry of head (*0–3 months*).

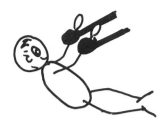

Fig. 6.49 Head lag (*0–3 months*).

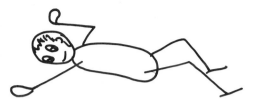

Fig. 6.50 Asymmetrical postures (*0–3 months*).

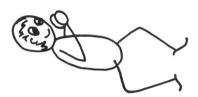

Fig. 6.51 Head, hands in midline (*4 months*).

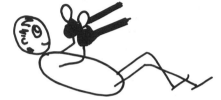

Fig. 6.52 Decrease head lag. Lifts head when about to be pulled up (*3–6 months*).

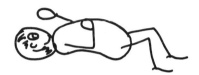

Fig. 6.53 Bridging hips (*5 months*).

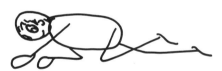

Fig. 6.54 Roll over (*6 months*).

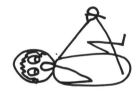

Fig. 6.55 Grasp feet (*7 months*).

Fig. 6.56 Lying straight, symmetry (*8 months*).

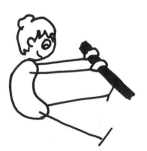

Fig. 6.57 Pull self to sitting. Dislikes supine (*9–12 months*).

Treatment suggestions and daily care for all levels of development

Supine rise to sitting and development of head righting (rising)

From 0–6 months normal development level   Help the child *to overcome head lag* using all or some of the following suggestions:

1   First have the child lying half-way down against a back support, or cushions and encourage him to come up to sitting. Gradually decrease the back support so that eventually he raises his head and trunk from supine to sitting.

2   At first you will also have to hold his shoulders well forward, then later his upper arms and, as soon as possible, have him grasp your hands with his elbows straight. In these ways pull the child up to sitting, *waiting* for his own active head raise and later head and trunk (righting) raising. Some children bring their heads up first, their trunks follow. In others trunks may come up first and stimulate the head next (Head-on-body righting; Body-on-head righting).

Carry out (1) and (2) slowly from supine or half-lying to sitting and lower the child back from sitting to supine.

3   Many children manage to raise their heads if pulled to sitting in diagonal directions and, only later, can accomplish this coming straight up from supine to sitting. This diagonal direction is often preferable, as this is how the child will pull himself to sitting. This is seen in normal motor development at about 9 months.

4   Pull the child's shoulder or arm diagonally across her body to the opposite side (Fig. 6.58). Help her rotate her body and lift her head as she is brought up to sitting. As the child comes up to sitting she may automatically lean on her forearm and may require help to take weight onto this forearm. If she cannot use her forearm, for support, you may hold both her hands, arms or shoulders and pull them across and over to one side of her body as she comes up to sitting in this diagonal direction.

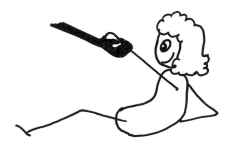

Fig. 6.58 Supine rise to sitting.

Note   In using methods 1–4 the child's legs should be observed as he rises to sitting. If his legs stretch, press together or twist inwards, then hold them apart, turn them outward on either side of a wedge, cushion or your knee or forearm (Fig. 6.59).

The child's arms should be held straight at the elbows and turned outward if there is a strong tendency for his arms to twist inwards from the shoulders or bend tightly to his body.

Children who bend their knees excessively after the normal level of 3 months, and children who have tight hamstrings may have them stretched by the therapist or by knee-pieces during these rising reactions.

5   Rising to sitting may also be trained from the side-lying position, particularly in those children who are excessively extended in the supine

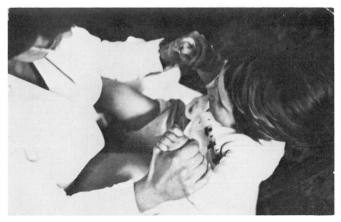

Fig. 6.59 Rising to sitting with the child's legs on either side of the therapist.

position, have very poor head raising from supine, or require additional activity of the shoulder girdle muscles, back extensors, or arm elevation pattern (Fig. 6.60). Child in side-lying, hips and knees semiflexed, head forward and arm underneath the head with bent elbow. Lift the child's upper arm behind his occiput, turn the arm outward from the shoulder and gently pull this arm and thus the child up toward side-sitting, lean on elbow. Wait for his own active participation as he responds to gently pulling him up towards sitting. Later let him rise to side-sitting, lean on his hand instead of on his elbow. Check that his palm is down on the ground, his head is lifted up and sideways and his back is rotated and extended.

From 6–10 months normal developmental level Help the child *to rise* to sitting on his own in the following ways:

1 Encourage his own head raise in supine by suspending him over the edge of a roll, your lap, a bed or a large ball. At first hold the child behind his shoulders, also place bells or toys on his tummy or feet so that the child is motivated to look up at them or at his toes (painted red if necessary!). Later, let him hang down over the edge of your lap, or the roll, and rock him upside down and call to him to raise his head.

2 Supine to sitting should be carried out by helping the child to grasp a rope, parallel bars or vertical bars with one hand across his body, and pull himself to sitting in a diagonal direction with half-rotation of his trunk.

3 Supine to sitting can be accomplished by the child if he holds a short pole or stick, held by you as well, with help to sitting. Do not let him hunch his shoulders and excessively bend elbows and wrists to do this.

Remember the normal child will first come up to sitting from supine in a diagonal direction with a half-roll to one side and lean on one elbow or hand. He will only come straight up to sitting from supine much later, as this is an adult pattern seen in normal children over 4 years. Normally the child at the developmental level of 6–10 months may also roll over and rise to sitting. Rolling should also be trained for this.

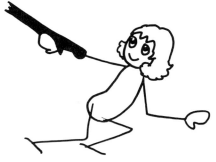

Fig. 6.60 Rising to sitting from side-lying.

Physiotherapy suggestions for rolling and roll-and-rise

Rolling techniques will help the child to roll to side-lying where his hands might meet and he can see them. Correct rolling methods correct the abnormal positions of the legs and arms and can also stimulate head righting, decrease infantile neck righting and stimulate various body derotative and rotative reflexes, and so learn to roll over to rise. He is then, in effect, using his body rotative reflexes for rising from supine. Some children need rolling for locomotion and exploring space. Some of the many methods available are:

Reflex rolling or primitive reactions Turn the baby or child's head to one side and hold his jaw firmly. Press down and across the fifth intercostal space towards the *opposite* side. A reflex rotation will begin at the pelvis causing both knees and then one knee to flex up and over to the side of the child's occiput. This technique initiates rolling and prepares for 'roll-and-rise', also actively corrects leg adduction-extension, arm flexion, hand fisting and abnormal 'roll-en-masse' (Fig. 6.61).

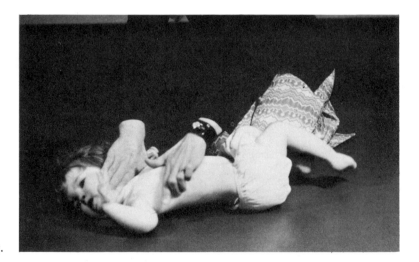

Fig. 6.61 Reflex rolling.

Side-lying Rotate the child's shoulder girdle forward while rotating his pelvis back. Change to rotation of the shoulder backward and pelvis forward, and vice versa (Figs 6.62, 6.63). If speed is correct and the rotary stretch on the trunk adequate, these 'counter rotations' stimulate an active response in the child's shoulder or pelvis or in both areas. This also treats the rolling 'in one piece' as seen say, in the neck righting reaction. If rotation of the shoulder girdle is possible against some manual resistance, there is often an associated head raising with the rotation. Rotation of the girdles pelvic/shoulder not only facilitates rolling but also initiates arm movements and leg movements. Train shoulder rotation backwards as a

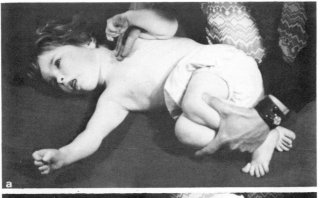

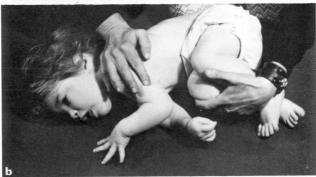

Fig. 6.62 a,b, Using knees to rotate pelvis in side-lying.

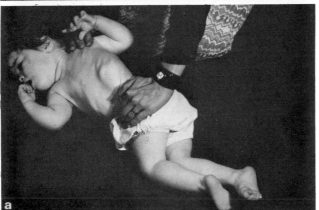

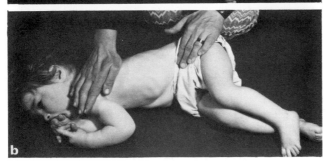

Fig. 6.63 Rotation of the shoulder girdles and pelvic girdles.

preliminary to pulling the arm out from underneath the body in those children who get their arm caught in rolling over.

Supine. Leg patterns

1 Bend both the child's knees across to the opposite side whilst rotating and holding his upper shoulder back. Release his shoulders and an active roll of the upper trunk follows. This roll might be manually resisted at the shoulder as well, but check that correct resistance is given so that a full flexion spasm does *not* occur (Fig. 6.62).

2 Stretch one of the child's legs into extension-abduction and then stimulate this leg to move to flexion-adduction to the opposite side. Wait for his upper trunk to roll over bringing the arm across (Fig. 6.64). A retraction of the shoulder often delays or even prevents the arm coming over within the child's roll from supine to prone. If possible facilitate leg flexion-adduction against resistance given at the knee and thigh.

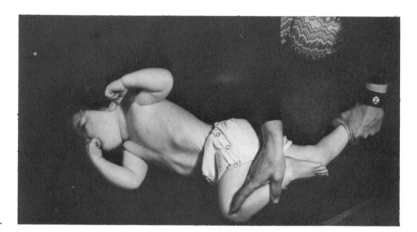

Fig. 6.64 Supine, leg patterns.

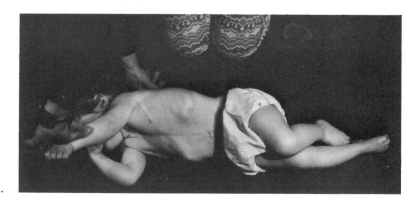

Fig. 6.65 Supine, arm patterns.

Arm patterns

1 Bring the child's arm from his side in shoulder extension-abduction-internal rotation and across his body to flexion-adduction-external rotation (child's palm must be towards his face) (Fig. 6.65). This stimulates the roll of his head, trunk and legs. The therapist may carry this out passively, use stretch and resistance or motivate a baby to reach for a toy on the opposite side of the moving arm.

2 Elevate and hold both the child's arms above his head in supine or in prone. Bring one arm across to the other to stimulate the child's automatic roll.

Note

1 Prone-supine rolling-use the arm or leg pattern of extension-rotation.

2 During rolling over, various leg patterns are themselves stimulated i.e. leg flexes over with the roll from supine to prone in some children. In others the child may use the leg to 'push-off' in an extended-abducted pattern (Fig. 6.66). During the roll from prone to supine, some children extend and abduct the upper leg. Other children flex the upper leg as they roll. Similarly arm patterns vary. The therapist must select the technique according to the reaction she wishes to obtain.

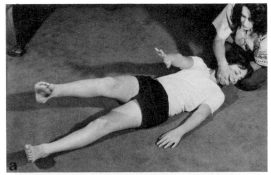

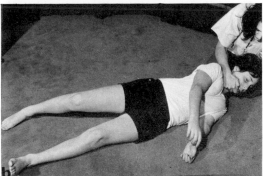

Fig. 6.66 a, b, Head pattern to stimulate rolling. *Note* limb reaction a, b.

3   Combinations of head, arm and leg patterns also vary.

Head patterns   Raise the child's head into flexion-rotation and wait for him to follow with rolling towards the side to which his face is rotated. Hold his head lightly as he rolls. You may have to hold his chin up as he reaches prone. Resisted head flexion-rotation may be used as well in children who have good head control and respond with rolling in their waist and not en-masse. Prone to supine rolling is carried out with head raise to extension-rotation. The arm patterns above may also provoke the head patterns. Some children may use an arm to 'push-off' together with head patterns (Fig. 6.66).

Rolling to instructions   *Head, arm or leg* patterns may be carried over from the facilitation techniques by some intelligent children. Instructions used

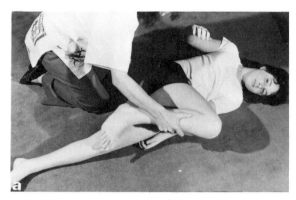

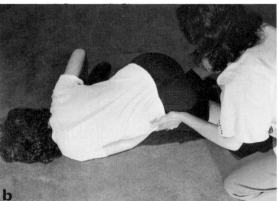

Fig. 6.67 a, b. Roll-to-rise onto hands and knees. *Note* many methods exist for this but must be demonstrated clinically.

for say: *prone lying* with arms overhead 'lift your head and one (right) arm up and back as far as possible', 'roll over'; 'lift your leg up and back, over to the other side', 'roll over'.

supine lying 'Bend one knee right across to the other side as far as it will go', 'roll over', 'grasp your hands and stretch your elbows—bring both arms over to one side as far as possible', 'roll over'; 'lift your head and look over to one side as far as possible', 'roll over'.

Treatment suggestions and daily care

Rolling

1   Place the child on his back, on his side or on his stomach (with face and neck over the edge) on a blanket. Hold each end of the blanket—two adults may be needed, and suspend the child in the blanket just off the ground. Tip the child gently from side to side, waiting for him to complete his roll over. If he cannot do this himself you can roll him in the blanket until he 'picks up' the rolling motion himself. *Do not* do this with a child who arches his back or overextends when in prone position. Keep repeating this roll sideways in suspension in supine with his head, shoulders and hips bent. Also suspend the child in a hammock, if arching persists in supine position.
2   Child lying on his back—bend one hip and knee well over to the opposite side and wait for him to complete the roll over (Fig. 6.64).
3   Bring one of his arms over to the opposite side with the palm of his hand towards his face, or offer him a toy he likes on the opposite side, this may lead to a roll over (Fig. 6.65).
4   Child lying on his stomach—bring his hip and pelvis, or his shoulders, back and towards the opposite side and encourage rolling. Some children may push off on one hand to help roll from prone to supine.
5   Child in prone or supine on a soft thick sponge rubber mattress or inflatable bed. Press down on one side of his body so that he tips over towards you and rolls. Rolling on such surfaces is often easier as he does not get 'stuck' with his arm caught under his body. At first it is necessary to place the arm, which gets caught underneath, above his head.
6   Encourage rolling on all surfaces, floors, carpets, grass and sand. Make an incline with a pile of mattresses or sponge rubber, or place the child on the top of a slight mound of grass or sand and let gravity help him roll downhill on his own.
7   If a child can roll over *wait* for him to do so. In addition train him to roll over from his back to his stomach and get up onto his hands and knees as described in Prone Development, 3–6 months level or Fig. 6.67 a,b).

STAGES IN SUPINE DEVELOPMENT

0–3 MONTHS NORMAL DEVELOPMENTAL LEVEL

Common problems

Delay in gradual overcoming of head lag on pull to sitting.

Abnormal performance (Fig. 6.68)   Opisthotonus, or excessive extension of either head, shoulder girdle retraction, back and legs or all of them. Some arch into opisthotonus in infancy but become floppy later. Floppy babies may have intermittent extensor spasms of head, spine and hips. They may also lie in 'frog' positions with the legs flexed-abducted-externally rotated, arms limp at their sides or in shoulder abduction, elbow flexion, hands open or closed. Apparently normal flexion positions may also be present in babies who later become spastics. Kicking of legs begins but may be simultaneous with abnormal asymmetry in that one leg flexes, abducts and sometimes externally rotates, while the other flexes adducts and sometimes internally rotates, or one may kick more vigorously than the other. This asymmetry may become so great that the legs look 'windswept' to one side, especially when kicking stops. Hip dislocation is threatening in the adducted-internally rotated leg. Persistent head turning to one side may occur.

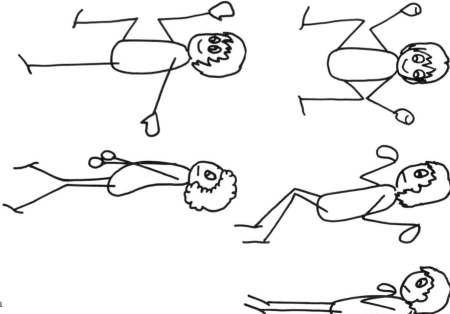

Fig. 6.68   Some abnormal patterns in supine.

Reflex reactions Normally these include grasp reflex, Moro reaction, asymmetrical tonic neck reaction, leg crossed extensor reflex, withdrawal reflex, neck righting reaction. On passively pulling the child to sitting, his legs should flex-adduct and, by the next 3–6 months level, flex-abduct. A response of extension-adduction of the legs is abnormal. Some cerebral palsied children even extend the hips so much that their hips come well off the surface.

Treatment suggestions and daily care

1 *See* rising to sitting, head raising and rolling techniques (pp. 96–103).
2 Bring the child's arms well forward and turn them out from his shoulders, so that both hands touch your face, or make him touch his own hands, mouth, chest or abdomen naming these body parts. Stimulate visually and with noises in the centre to encourage his head holding in the centre and hands should make contact with bells or musical toys dangling in the midline.
3 Eye-to-eye contact with your eyes parallel to his, at first in the centre. Then stimulate him to follow sounds, lights and mobiles from side-to-side (see Hand Function, page 184).

Physiotherapy suggestions

Abnormal reflex reactions and abnormal performance
1 *Discourage* supine if the child has asymmetrical tonic neck reaction after 4 months; excessive Moro after 6 months or has extensor spasms. It is better that the child is in prone or sitting positions selected according to his level of development. Head should be in the centre and both arms held parallel and forward at the shoulder level in these positions. If supine is inevitable during periods in the day, hold the child's head up into flexion in the hollow of a large cushion; use a hammock (Fig. 6.69). This overcomes the head falling or pressing back into extension. Head flexion often diminishes the A.T.N.R., Moro or extensor thrusts. In this position hold his arms symmetrical (parallel) and brought well (flexed) forward at the shoulders. Motivate these symmetrical arm movements with toys, mobiles and so on.
2 Excessively extended children should be flexed at head and shoulders, and hips in side-lying or supine (Fig. 6.69). The severely extended child, especially if the arms are always at the sides with retracted shoulders and bent elbows, should be kept in side-lying with support from pillows or a 'side-lying board' (Fig. 6.69) so that his hands will be able to meet and so that he can see them, so that they can touch his mouth and later reach for toys in front of him (5 months' level). Place a toy between his hands that can easily be grasped (see Hand Function), later train him to lie on his side alone. Show the child how to balance in side-lying with one leg on top of the other, as well as one in front of the other.

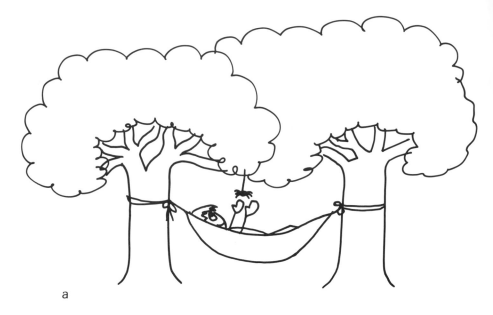

a

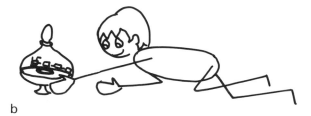

Fig. 6.69 Some corrective positions.

b

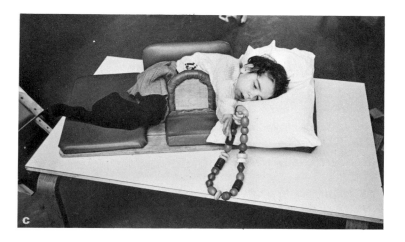

3 For a child with abnormally straight legs, pressed together and turned in, use abduction pants. For 'frog position' use sandbags to keep the legs together as you train rising or sitting or talk to the child in supine. Pants that are well stitched down the centre can be used to bring the legs together in lying. Sometimes arms held down and in front stimulate legs coming together.

4 Persistent head turning should be discouraged by getting the child to look the other way. His bed should be on the opposite side of the room, offer toys, communication and even food from the side towards which the child rarely turns. Carry the child so that he can also look to the side which is not usually preferred.

The physiotherapist must check that the child does not have a torticollis which requires stretching or even an operation. Plagiocephaly may accompany head turning. This strong head turning or preference has been observed in some babies who were really normal (Robson).

5 See therapy for grasp reflex in Hand Function (p. 188), Moro in the Development of Sitting (p. 120), crossed extensor reflex, withdrawal reflex, in Development of Standing (p. 149), neck righting reflex in Rolling Techniques (p. 98).

6 Abnormal synergies, i.e. leg extension-adduction-internal rotation are best corrected in the creeping patterns at this level in prone development. If prone development is not indicated in the particular child, train reciprocal leg movement in supine. Carry out active assisted full range of reciprocal motion. Hold the child's knees and bend one hip and knee up and out, holding the other leg straight and turned out. Change the motion by bringing the bent leg down as you move the straight leg up into flexion (Fig. 6.70).

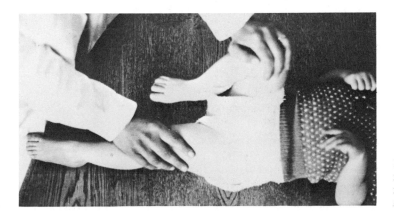

Fig. 6.70 Assisted active reciprocal motion. Hold one leg well down while fully flexing the other. Point knees outward.

4–6 MONTHS NORMAL DEVELOPMENT LEVEL

Common problems

Delay in acquisition of symmetry, in keeping head in the centre, in bringing the arms together and in 'hand regard'. Delay in the disappearance of head lag and in acquiring ability to raise the head off the bed. The child is unable to 'bridge' his hips off the floor, unable to reach for a toy (see Hand Function, p. 185).

Abnormal performance   Flexed legs now abnormally extend-adduct and internally rotate in many spastics in lying supine and when brought from supine to sitting position. Normally legs flex-abduct and externally rotate at this level. Presence of clenched hands. Abnormal absence of isolated foot movements or knee movements, as these only occur as part of 'mass patterns'.

Reflex reactions   May not be developing body derotation. Reflexes of 0–6 months level may not be disappearing.

Treatment suggestions and daily care

1   See Hand Function (p. 185).
2   See rise up to sitting and rolling techniques (p. 98), especially rolling with rotation or turning at the child's waist line during a roll over.

Physiotherapy suggestions

Arm reach   Child in side-lying and progress to supine. Facilitate arm patterns of flexion-adduction-external rotation with straight elbow and also with bent elbow, so that hands touch the child's mouth. Carry this out as a unilateral pattern in side-lying and as a bilateral pattern in supine (see Hand Function, Fig. 6.186, p. 175).

Bridging   Hold the child's feet flat on the floor. He raises his hips to let a toy go 'under the bridge'. Check that this is not done by using a lumbar lordosis. Check that arms do not flex up into abnormal postures. Hold the 'bridge' steady while the wind tries to 'blow it over'. On this instruction the therapist gives manual resistance at the side of the child's pelvis, or on the anterior superior iliac spines, or one hand in front and one behind to rotate his pelvis. The child must maintain the stability of 'the bridge' as far as possible. A pillow under his hips may help initially as he learns to maintain control against your manual pressure and resistance.

Note Semi-bridging and moving backwards is a form of locomotion used by some athetoids and more rarely by spastics. However, this is often abnormal as it includes excessive hypertonic arching in the head and back and retraction of the shoulder. This should be discouraged and another form of locomotion offered to the child.

6–9 MONTHS NORMAL MOTOR DEVELOPMENTAL LEVEL

Common problems

Delay in grasping feet with legs in the air. The child is unable to roll over or pull himself towards sitting.

Abnormal performance He cannot lie straight with arms and legs extended or with legs abducted-extended-externally rotated. A variety of abnormal postures may be seen including asymmetry of head, trunk or limbs or all of these. Normally, the pull-to-sit should provoke extension-abduction of legs.

Abnormal rolling patterns may be roll, leading with head and arms but with legs stiff and straight or passive; roll, using legs but upper arm bent and retracted at the shoulder; roll, using a 'flexion into a ball', or using an arching of the back and head to roll over. No rotation at the child's waist (body rotative reactions) i.e. either rolling in one piece or using the abnormal total flexion or extension; roll to one side only, in say hemiplegia, towards the affected side only, using the unaffected side to carry out the roll over, or in say quadriplegia using the less affected side to carry out the roll, or in others, simply being unable to roll to a particular side.

Treatment suggestions and daily care

1   See, rising to sitting, 6–10 months level, Rolling Techniques (p. 98) and Hand Function (p. 189) (Figs. 6.71, 6.72).
2   Have the child in supine and help him to hold one or both of his feet. Turn his hips and knees outward and bend his leg so his foot is touching his hand. Gently stretch his knee and lift his leg so that he can reach for, look at and also grasp his feet and hold them. First bend his hips and lift his bottom off the bed if he is unable to reach. The child must also actively bend his hip and knee to his chest so that the full hip flexion is attained. Ask him to 'kiss his knee', 'to pull his sock or shoe off his toes' or to 'hug his knees to his chest'.

Note No further developmental training is needed in supine as, from 10 months' onward the child normally *dislikes* lying supine and persists in rolling out of this position or pulling up to sitting.

3   Having trained the child to rise from supine to sitting *does not mean he can sit*. See Development of Sitting (p. 111) which should be trained at the same time as Supine Development. Levels of development of sitting and rise to sitting may be at different motor ages.

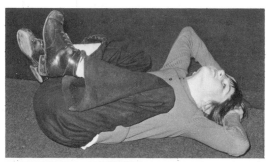

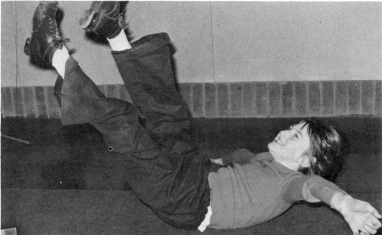

Fig. 6.71 Athetoid girl using her own method of rising (bend knees to chest and swing up to sitting, or grasp clothes and pull up to sitting).

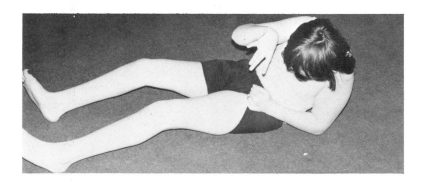

Fig. 6.72 Spastic boy using his own method of rising to sitting. He grasps his clothes and pulls himself up alone.

DEVELOPMENT OF SITTING

The following main aspects should be developed:

Postural fixation of the head or vertical head control. Normally developed by 3 months.

Head righting or rising to the vertical position. Normally developed by 3 months.

Postural fixation of the head and the trunk (Fig. 6.73)   Normally developed 3–6 months and independent by 9 months.

Head and trunk righting or rising from sitting, leaning or slumped forward, backward or sideways, to upright sitting (Fig. 6.74)   Normally developed between 3–12 months depending upon the positions and support given to the child.

Note   Rising to sitting from supine see Supine Development (p. 95) and from prone see Prone Development (p. 72). Rising from sitting to standing, see Development of Standing and walking (p. 137).

Postural fixation of the shoulder girdle   Normally developed 3–6 months. This is associated with a reinforcement of fixation of the head and also with the use of the arms for supports in sitting.

Postural fixation of head on trunk and trunk on pelvis. Normally developed by 6 months with support and independently with head and trunk by 9 months.

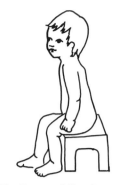

Fig. 6.73   Postural fixation.

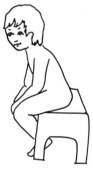

Fig. 6.74   Rising to upright sitting and reverse

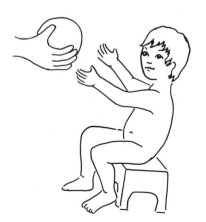

Fig. 6.75   Counterpoising.

Sitting counterpoising head, arm, trunk and leg movements (Fig. 6.75). Normally developed 6–12 months (see also Development of Hand Function, p. 170, Dressing and Feeding, p. 194).

Tilt reactions (Fig. 6.76)   When the child is tilted sideways, forwards or backwards (his bottom is tilted off the horizontal). Normally developed by 9–12 months.

Saving reactions and propping reactions if the child falls. Normally developed forward about 5–7 months, sideways about 9 months and backward about 12 months.

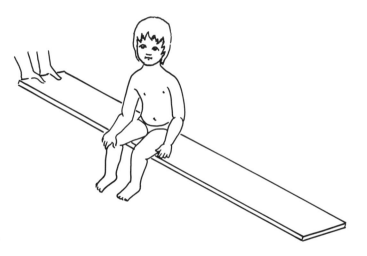

Fig. 6.76   Tilt reaction.

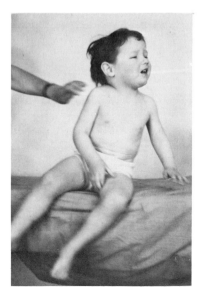

Fig. 6.77   Saving reactions in the arms and legs.

STAGES IN DEVELOPMENT OF SITTING (Figs. 6.78–6.91)

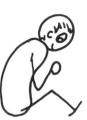

Fig. 6.78 Sitting head uncontrolled, flexion in total child (*0–3 months*).

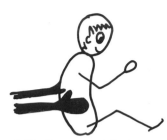

Fig. 6.79 Decrease of flexion, vertical head control develops (*0–3 months*).

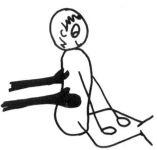

Fig. 6.80 Sitting lean on hands, flattening of upper back develops lumbar kyphosis still present (*4–6 months*).

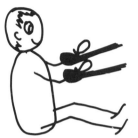

Fig. 6.81 Sitting with less support, back straighter, legs straighter, turning out and apart (*4–6 months*).

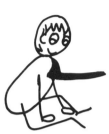

Fig. 6.82 Sitting lean on elbows, hips flexed-abducted-externally rotated. Less support and without support (*4–6 months*).

Fig. 6.83 Sitting in baby chair with back and sides supporting or propped on a pillow support (*4–6 months*).

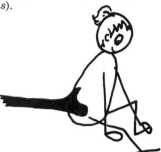

Fig. 6.84 Sitting lean on hands and lift one hand to play, with feet or a toy (*6–9 months*).

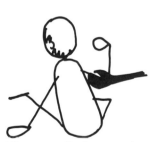

Fig. 6.85 Saving reactions and propping in arms (*6–9 months*).

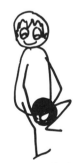

Fig. 6.86 Sitting alone on the ground (*6–9 months*).

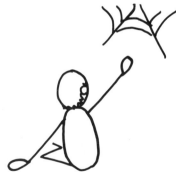

Fig. 6.87 Sitting reach in all directions, hand support (*6–9 months*).

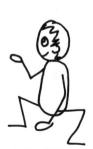

Fig. 6.88 Sitting turn to play, reach, no hand support (*9–12 months*).

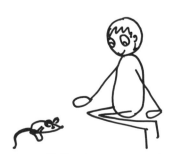

Fig. 6.89 Sitting in various positions (*9–12 months*).

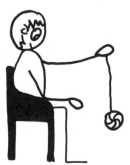

Fig. 6.90 Sitting in a chair and play, sit alone in regular chair on a stool (*9–12 months*).

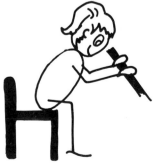

Fig. 6.91 Rising out of sitting and getting to sitting positions (*9–12 months*).

ABNORMAL POSTURES IN SITTING AT ALL LEVELS OF DEVELOPMENT (Fig. 6.92)

These may be due to:

1   Absence of the above postural mechanisms and compensatory abnormal postures to obtain balance.
2   Presence of hypertonus.
3   Attempts by an older child to control disrupting involuntary movements.
4   Use of incorrect size and type of chairs, tables, pushchairs, wheelchairs and continual placement of the child in only one or more poor sitting positions.

Absence of postural fixation is associated with falling backwards or leaning backward (sliding out of the seat of the chair). The abnormal postures may arise in compensation for this as follows:

1   Head and trunk flex although hips remain extended beyond the right angle which is normally seen between hips and trunk. Postural fixation at the hip is absent (Fig. 6.92, b, c).
2   Head may hyperextend, or chin may jut forward to prevent overflexion forward of the trunk and falling forward in overcompensation (Fig. 6.92, b).
3   Arms may be held up in the air, elbows straight, shoulder hunched and

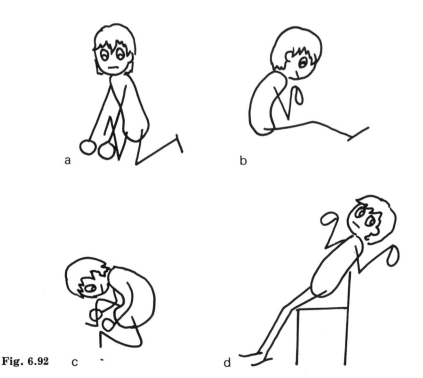

Fig. 6.92

flexed at 45–90° forward, as if the arms are counterbalancing the backward lean.

4 Arms may be held up in the air at the sides in abduction with elbow flexion, shoulders hunched, retracted or protracted (Fig. 6.92, d).

5 Arms may be held tensely flexed at shoulders, elbows and hands as the child grasps a support near his body (Fig. 6.92, b). Grasping a support may also be carried out in other patterns such as shoulder flexion, elbow extension and inward rotation of the arms (Fig. 6.92, a). The total abnormal sitting posture may be maintained with or without grasping a support to prevent falling.

6 Legs not only semi-extend beyond the right angle at the hip, but also adduct-internally rotate with extended knees and sometimes feet, or the hips adduct, internally rotate with the knees flexing strongly over the edge of the chair. If the 'grasping' of the edge of the chair is inadequate to maintain sitting, the child's legs also twist around the legs of the chair. If the chair is too high or the child is sitting on a bed or table the hip adduction-internal rotation occurs with legs hanging over the edge. This is particularly precarious and any of the above postures increase to preserve balance. Feet may plantarflex to reach the ground for support or if the ground is near enough feet are held in planovalgus as an extra base for sitting balance.

7 Sitting on the floor with his bottom between his feet and his legs internally rotated and bent at the knee, is often seen in cerebral palsied children as this is one way in which the unstable pelvis can be fixed. Some children also need to lean on their hands on clenched fists with arms turned in to support an unstable trunk and shoulder girdle. Others develop head and trunk postural fixation in this position. Although this posture is seen in normal children, it is not held for the many long periods of time as in the abnormal child. Deformities of the hip joints, knee flexion contractures and foot deformities may be developed in this position unless it can be varied with other postures (Fig. 6.92, a).

Tailor-sitting, long-sitting on the floor with legs straight in front and sitting on a chair may be carried out with a very round back and sacral sitting as there is inadequate postural fixation of the pelvis on the trunk to obtain the normal right angle at the hips and a straight back.

8 Some children acquire better postural fixation on one side of their bodies than on the other and may tend to sit more on one buttock. This is most obvious in hemiplegics. Scoliosis may result from this asymmetrical weight distribution.

Abnormal sitting postures in spastic (hypertonic) children

If the child is also hypertonic, he will assume the same postures already described, but the shortened or shortening spastic or rigid muscles maintain or create these abnormal postures, as well as others. Thus prolonged sitting in any one position is particularly dangerous as it causes deformity and so disabling influences on the development of standing and walking.

The above postures associated with the tightness of spastic muscles will be seen as:

1 Stiff extension so that the child cannot be flexed into the sitting position unless special methods are used. Some children can overcome their 'extensor thrusts' or extensor hypertonus by using flexor hypertonus and sitting in excessive flexion.

2 Some severely extended children may collapse into a flexion spasm or flexion and floppiness once the extensor hypertonus or spasm is overcome by the therapist. No sitting is possible in either position.

3 Most children achieve a position somewhere between full flexion or extension. The falling backward and extensor thrust seems to remain *in the hips* but trunk flexes with arms and head extends, legs assume various postures depending on the distribution of the spasticity in each child. Trunk, head and arms also vary according to the child. Some children have hypertonus in the trunk, often on one side only. Scoliosis together with torticollis may be present.

4 Tight hamstrings are often present in hypertonic children. The pelvis is tilted back in sitting by the pull of the tight hamstrings. If the knees are extended as in long-sitting on the floor (Fig. 6.92, b) the child may fall backward as his hamstrings—do not allow this full extension. Many children can maintain long-sit with their pelvis tipped back in sacral sitting with a round back if they semiflex at the knees. On a chair, the child's knees can bend fully and this often tips the pelvis back into position for upright sitting with the child's weight on his tuberosities and not on his sacrum.

Knee flexion deformities are particularly threatening in these children especially if they have prolonged sitting on chairs, where they find sitting so much easier.

TREATMENT SUGGESTIONS AND DAILY CARE AT ALL LEVELS OF DEVELOPMENT

Practical points

Check

1 Abnormal posture.
2 Support given in Figs. 6.93–6.108.

1 Abnormal postures are corrected during all the methods. Special corrections may be given in addition for:

Kyphosis Use arm patterns involving elevation, as well as the general development of postural fixation of head, trunk and pelvis in sitting and other channels of development (see Arm patterns, p. 172).

Scoliosis Make sure the child sits on both his buttocks. Reaching overhead is helpful on the side of the concavity. Attach pad, behind and at the side of his shoulder, to his chair, to hold him upright. Sandbags or a roll of towels on his table under his forearm on the side of the concavity, or under the buttock on either the side of the concavity or convexity, should be tried to discover which props him into a more upright position.

Abnormal postures of arms, trunk, head, legs are often corrected at the same time if the child sits on *both* his ischial tuberosities, leans forward from his hips, leans on his open hands with elbows held straight. Legs should be held apart and turned outward. When knees are always in flexion, then use knee gaiters and sitting on or just off the floor if his back rounds, in preference to chair sitting. Feet should be flat on the ground if the child sits on a chair. Foot supports are essential if he is on a high chair. Correction of equinus feet, as discussed in Chapter 8, is important as this provides plantigrade feet as extra supports for sitting balance.

There are many modifications required according to each child's problems.

Some ideas to correct leg postures include sitting with legs apart and turned out on either side of large toys, a box of toys, bowl of sand or water, a small drum, straddling rolls, soft toys, the corner of the bed or chair, and across your hip or thigh. Do not have the child straddle anything of too great a diameter as he then increases hip internal rotation with excessive abduction of his hips. Abduction pants may have to be worn during sitting for better hip posture (Chapter 8). Tailor-sitting or side-sitting are preferable to sitting between his knees (Fig. 6.124), but should also be avoided if there is too much flexion in the child's hips and knees as well as abnormal adduction and internal rotation. Feet must also be checked in case they deform in these sitting positions.

Avoid prolonged sitting especially if there is tightness of hip and knee flexors. Encourage standing up and standing positions or prone lying instead.

Excessive hip, trunk and head extension is corrected within the postures above, as well as having the child learn to sit on low chairs, kneel sit (Fig. 6.110), sit in the corner of the sofa, or room, and into various sitting apparatus (see below). Carry the child in full flexion, to counteract severe extension and just before he is placed into his special 'flexion chairs'—see below and Fig. 7.8.

Remember that when the child leans forward from his hips to reach his toys, feet or prop himself on his hands, he should lean from his hip joint. He should not round his back instead of flexing in his hip. Help him by pressing your hand on the small of his back, if he cannot manage alone. Also make sure that the pull of tight hamstrings is not causing this and that a small raise onto a platform for his floor seat, is required. This is especially necessary if he is wearing knee extension splints. Sitting on a thick cushion or sponge on the floor, may also improve posture of his back.
CORRECT CHAIRS AND TABLES ALSO COUNTERACT ABNORMAL POSTURES.

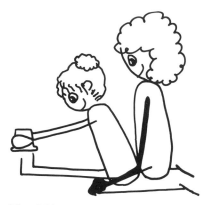

Fig. 6.93

2. Support   The methods suggested below are used for each level of development provided that the *appropriate amount* of support is given to the child (Figs 6.93–6.108).

Support is at first given to the child's shoulders so that his total body is supported, and he should only achieve vertical head control (0–3 months level). Holding his upper arms and using shoulder girdle fixation may act as a support to the whole child and also facilitate head control at the first level of sitting development. With further training support may be lowered to the child's body and waist (3–6 months level) and then to his hips and thighs (6–9 months level) sometimes to his feet only, and finally removed at the 7–9 months level when sitting alone is normally expected.

Note (a)   All methods may be used for sitting on the floor and on the child's chair. Sitting on the floor is emphasised in babies and young children whilst in older children at the same early developmental level, chair sitting is emphasised.

(*b*) Sitting on the child's chair may be achieved before sitting on the floor in athetoids, spastics with very tight hamstrings and any developmentally delayed children with particularly poor sitting balance. Stable feet held flat on the ground are an additional aid to sitting in a chair, but is of course, absent in sitting on the floor.

(*c*) Special chairs and equipment aid supported sitting at early (0–6 months) developmental levels. They should be removed when the child develops his own control. Thus 'cerebral palsy chairs' or wheelchairs are usually equivalent to sitting at a 6 months normal developmental level.

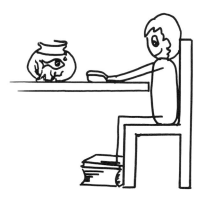

Fig. 6.94

Various methods of giving and reducing support are discussed below.

Support may be given with the adult's body against the child's back as he is held on her lap or the child sits across a roll with the adult sitting close behind him. The adult then moves her body away from the child's back and support is only given at his waist level or at his hips and thighs (Fig. 6.93).

The child may be supported in front or lean against a table edge, preferably padded, at his shoulder level and this support is lowered to waist level and finally removed so that he sits at the table without leaning against it by 9 months normal developmental level. Feet should be supported on a firm surface (Fig. 6.94).

The table may be used as a support together with the child grasping a horizontal pole attached to the table, the support of the table is removed and grasp alone can be used before total removal of table and grasp. The cut-out on the table offers more support at first, but should be removed as soon as possible (Fig. 6.95).

Whilst training sitting, the support at the child's chest may be given by the adult instead of by a table. The child may hold the adult's shoulders or

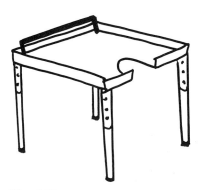

Fig. 6.95

one of her hands, whilst her other hand supports his chest, subsequently his waist and finally his thighs, knees or just his feet flat on the ground.

Hold shoulders forward for vertical head control. Encourage head hold in the midline with eye-to-eye contact. Move support down child's trunk for next developmental levels (Fig. 6.96).

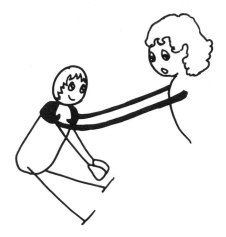

Fig. 6.96

Joint compression through head in vertical alignment with trunk *or* hold baby/child and bounce him on his bottom on sponge rubber, trampoline, inflatable toy, beach ball or your lap (Fig. 6.97). Check that head, trunk and bottom are in alignment. Use compression through head and or shoulders (Fig. 7.1) during feeding, play, communication, and similar activities.

Fig. 6.97

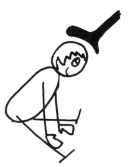

Child takes weight on forearms. (Fig. 6.98). If child presses his arms to his chest use a roll of towels or sponge wedge to avoid this. Joint compression through shoulders or head may also be used.

Child is helped to lean on his forearms into adult's hands (Fig. 6.99). Adult reinforces this joint compression by pushing child's upper arm into his shoulder joint. Head and trunk control is partially stimulated.

Visual and auditory stimuli at child's eye level for vertical head and trunk control in sitting (Fig. 6.100). Upright posture is encouraged. Correct chair to aid this is needed.

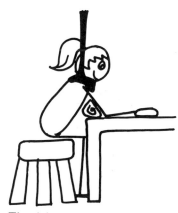

Fig. 6.98

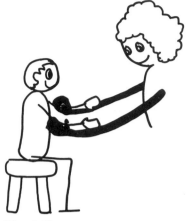

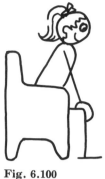

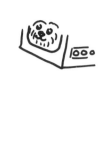

Fig. 6.99

Fig. 6.100

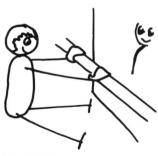

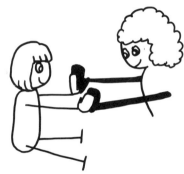

Fig. 6.101

Fig. 6.102

Sitting grasping a pole, edge of a table or adult's hands (Fig. 6.101). Elbows should be straight and symmetrical. The support may be grasped with his arms at shoulder level, below shoulder level or above shoulder level. Child leans against table edge at lower levels of development (0–6 months).

Child pushes his open hands against adult's hands with wrists dorsi-flexed (Fig. 6.102).

Child may also push against wall, make 'hand prints' on powdered or soaped mirror or push firm toy to make a sound (Fig. 6.103). Trunk support may be given by leaning against a table edge or manually at 0–6 months level.

Child leans on hands on floor, child on a chair can lean on his hands (Fig. 6.104).

Stimulate head righting by bringing his shoulders forward and then take his upper arms, turn them out and elevate them (Fig. 6.105). Arm raising to abduction-external rotation against manual resistance given at

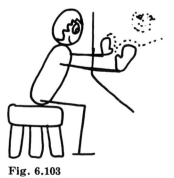

Fig. 6.103

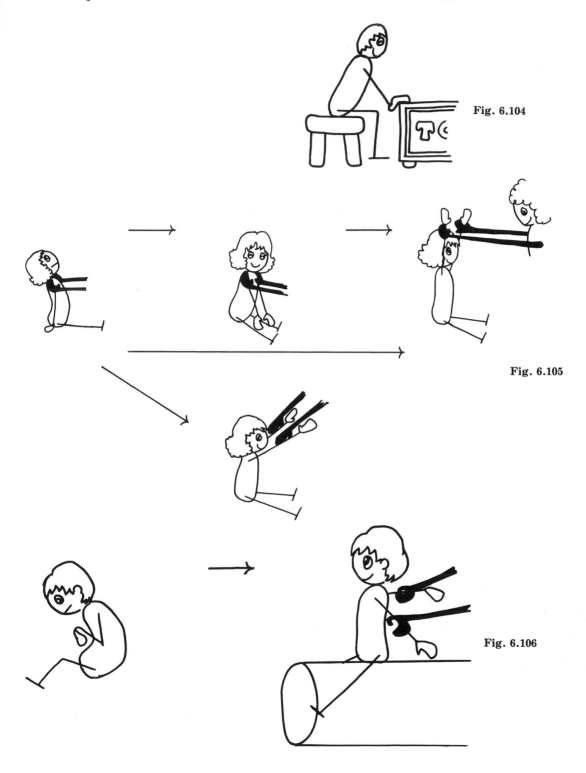

Fig. 6.104

Fig. 6.105

Fig. 6.106

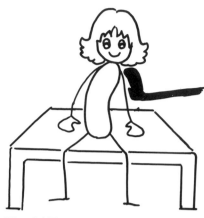

Fig. 6.107

the upper arm. (See Arm patterns, Correction of sitting posture, p. 121.)

Stimulate head righting by pulling shoulder girdle backwards or arms back (Fig. 6.106). Child may also push arms back against your hands.

Manual resistance may be given at the child's shoulder on its lateral aspect or anteroposterior aspect (Fig. 6.107). This reinforces head fixation, shoulder girdle fixation (stability). Do this also with the child leaning on forearms (Fig. 6.98), on hands (Fig. 6.97), or grasping a support.

Note   Give the correct amount of resistance so that abnormal reactions are not provoked.

Chairs and tables

These are selected according to the child's developmental level to:
1   Train sitting.
2   Correct abnormal postures.
3   Provide stimulation which is more available in the upright sitting position than in lying.
4   Develop hand function. This development is trained in prone and supine but must not be prevented from occurring in the *upright* position of *supported* sitting, if sitting alone is a developmental level beyond any particular child. Meanwhile training of sitting balance must continue and be associated with hand function as soon as possible. (See Hand Function and the Postural Mechanisms, p. 169.)
Regular chairs are used:
1   To increase development of sitting balance and independent good posture.
2   To develop hand function together with sitting balance.
3   To make standing up from sitting possible.

Measurements   If chairs are not of the correct measurements for the child they can obstruct the development of sitting, cause or increase abnormal postures and prevent hand function (Fig. 6.108). Only use an armrest if that support is needed. The back rest is 100° to seat. Table should be up to the height of child's waist or higher if he lacks trunk control. There should be a *large* area of work space.

If the chair is *too high* the child will find lack of foot support for his dangling feet disturbing to his poor sitting balance. Plantarflexed feet may become plantarflexion deformity. If the chair is *too wide* the child may take more weight on one side as he slumps to that side. The lateral lean or slumping decreases balance and may lead to scoliosis. Place rolls of towel, sponge-covered blocks, sandbags or magazines to decrease a chair which is too wide. The seat could be made to fit his buttocks. If the chair seat is *too small* the child may not be able to balance without support to his thighs. His feet may twist or curl around the chair legs in his efforts to balance. Deformity of his feet and of flexed, adducted internally rotated knees may

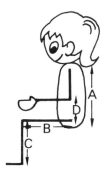

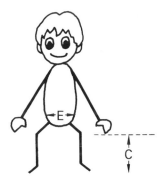

A   Height of backrest
B   Seat depth
C   Seat to floor
D   Armrest height
E   Seat width

Fig. 6.108

be encouraged. If the chair seat is *too long* he may slump backwards to the back support and increase hip extension, adduction and internal rotation, knee extension and plantarflexion or hip extension adduction, semiflexion of the knees and plantarflexion of his feet. Rounding of the back is inevitable. In all the above situations the child's hand function is made impossible or difficult.

Design of chairs for specific abnormal postures

Hip and knee adduction-internal rotation   Use one or two padded pommels or a roll as a seat or thigh straps (see Figs b.109–6.116). Correct hip extension, as this also corrects adduction-internal rotation.

Hip and knee extension, extensor thrusts and sliding out of the chair, sacral sitting, can be controlled by some or all of the following:
1   Increase the angle of the seat so that a 'jack-knife' position of the hips is obtained or place a roll of towel under the child's knees in a regular chair. The 'jack-knife' position may be as much as 45° to the back in severely extended children. For milder cases, use a small wedge on the chair or a wooden build-up (Figs 6.114, 6.117) to incline the seat backwards to prevent the child sliding forward or extending back during arm movements, especially arm elevation.
2   Raise the back of the chair for some children who continually go backwards.
3   Place the child well back in his chair and use thigh straps if he cannot maintain this position. The thigh straps must be nailed between the thighs

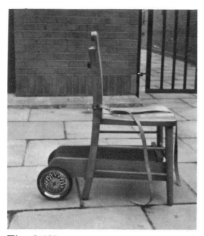

Fig. 6.109

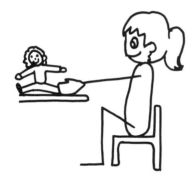

Fig. 6.110

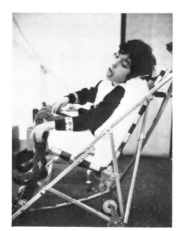

Fig. 6.111

at the groin so that the child is pulled well back against the backrest of the chair (Fig. 6.109). Use rubber tubing on the straps to prevent chafing.

4 Use a diagonal strap across their hips and preferably tied below the level of the seat. A padded pommel ($2\frac{1}{2}''$ dowel) may be helpful as well.

5 A deep canvas seat, a deep inflatable chair, sacks filled with polystyrene beads ('beanbag' chairs) or tyres may be useful.

6 Stabilise chair if child tips chair backwards. Make base from a box or have extended bars or skis from front to back legs of the chair.

7 Do not have hard surfaces against the child's occiput, buttock or forefoot if they provoke extensor thrusts.

8 In a regular chair the sliding and extension may be actively controlled by the child if he is told to keep his bottom against the back of his chair. In addition, use a low stool or chair to increase flexion (Fig. 6.110). Have the child lean forward *from the hips*, towards his table, to grasp a support or towards the play equipment, sand try or water trough on a stand, or gardens built up to the child's waist level. This independent control is always preferable if it can be achieved.

Foot deformities and involuntary movements   The child should keep his feet flat on the ground. If he thrusts back and tips the chair, increase the hip flexion or remove the stimulus on the forefoot. Using a footstool and pressing his heels down helps. Foot rests with skis, tying ankles to chair legs or using sandbags or foot straps, all help control of feet.

Trunk kyphosis, scoliosis, extensor thrusts may be so severe that moulds are required and have to be attached to the child's chair or wheelchair (Fig. 6.111) (see Scoliosis above). Use table height to correct kyphosis in milder cases. Correction of hips and arm posture also corrects trunk posture in chairs.

Head control   Avoid use of head supports if there is any ability in the child to hold his head up. Side supports to backrest are available to stop the head falling sideways. Orthopaedic collars are preferred by some therapists. Remember that:

1 The child must not collapse into flexion in any chair. His balance must be stimulated.

2 Control of the *hips and pelvis only* often improves trunk posture and balance, arm posture and use. The resulting trunk fixation from stabilised hips also improves head control in many children.

3 The chair should look as normal and be as comfortable as possible.

4 The chair should be close to the ground so that the child can push down on to his feet when he is nearly ready to pull up to standing. High chairs may be used so that the young child can join the family around the table. Footrests for high chairs become essential for balance, hand function and correct posture.

5 Check measurements and amount of support given by the chair. This changes as the child gets older and more adequate in sitting balance.

6 Chair and table heights should relate to one another. Avoid any chair-table designs which make it impossible for a child to join his friends at a large table or next to the communal table.

Floor seats Select the correct floor seat so that the young child can play with toys on the floor or join other children playing on the ground in play-groups, playgrounds or sandpits (Fig. 6.112 a).

1 A well padded pommel for adducted legs. Two small pommels may be used close together and gradually moved apart as the child develops more adduction. (A padded jam-tin nailed to the chair may suffice.)

2 Height of the back should be at shoulder level of the child if he tends to fall back or arch back when sitting. Occasionally the head may require a padded back support. Curve the chairback to prevent shoulders and back of the child arching into extension. See cylindrical chairs (Fig. 6.112 b).

3 Height of the back and sides of the floor seat should be cut down to the child's waist level as he acquires more head and trunk control. A square back may be used, as well as triangular and cylindrical ones.

4 The width of the chair should be such that the child does not slide from side to side. Pad up the sides with sponge or newspapers so that this does not occur. A canvas or inflatable seat allows the child to sink into his own area of support.

5 Seat of chair is measured from child's hips to his knees.

6 The floor seat may be placed on wheels for locomotion if the child requires this; it may be used in a toilet seat; it may be tied onto a sturdy adult chair next to the family table. A table can be fitted to it.

7 The floor seat may have to be raised off the floor for those children who have a very rounded back. The height of the floor seat off the floor should be tested to see whether the child's back straightens. If this does not occur, it is important to give him a table which is high enough for his arms to be elevated to that point where his back straightens. A small firm pillow or back

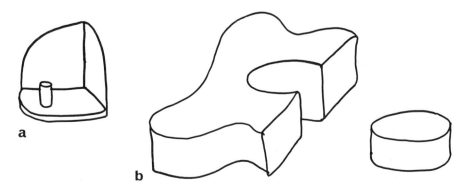

Fig. 6.112 Cylindrical chairs need not be cylindrical on the outside. Cushions can be put in for knee flexion.

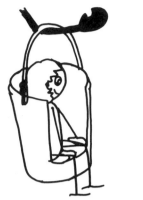

Fig. 6.113 Adapted bucket for sitting.

support may help to hold the back straight. Adjusting the position of the pommel (crutch support) may help. If none of these methods correct a severely rounded back then a *floor seat should not be used*.

Other equipment for sitting

1 Chair swings, back and sides on toy trucks, rocking horse or pedal cars. Inflatable chairs, baskets, plastic buckets or bins padded inside and cut out in front, boxes, carseats, cylinder packing cases, 'Safa' bath seat, Suzy bath seat and others help supported sitting. Children who extend or arch back can be held in sitting using some of this apparatus. However these seats *must* be stabilised near a wall or with weights. They may need a tray, table or low stool at the correct distance from the child so that he can use his hands (Figs 6.112–6.116).

Remember The child can grasp a horizontal bar to sit.
2 Toilet seats (Figs. 6.117–6.120). See also Chapter 7, Figs. 7.1, 7.2.
3 Push-chairs and wheelchairs (see Appendix).

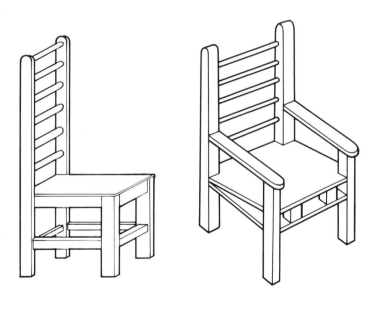

Fig. 6.114 Slatted back based on a design by Petö Institute. Child can sit sideways and hook his arm through slats for balance; use slats to push chair for walking aid. Stabilise base by using a box as base or skis attached. A box base also prevents legs twisting under the seat.

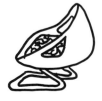

Fig. 6.115 Cosco seat with adjustable height.

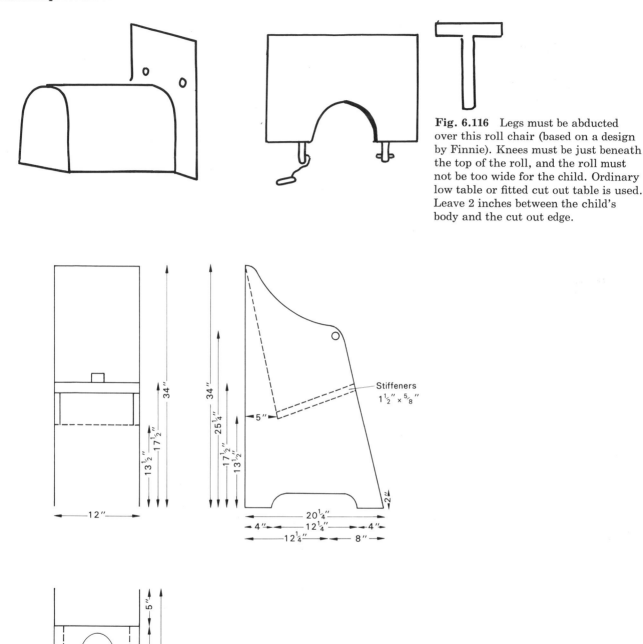

Fig. 6.116 Legs must be abducted over this roll chair (based on a design by Finnie). Knees must be just beneath the top of the roll, and the roll must not be too wide for the child. Ordinary low table or fitted cut out table is used. Leave 2 inches between the child's body and the cut out edge.

Stiffeners 1½″ × ⅝″

Scale 1 – 12

Timber ½″ (7mm) Plywood

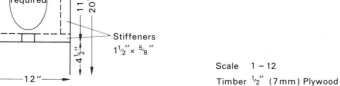

Fig. 6.117 Potty chair, cut hole out to shape of potty. Pad the back and sides of the chair with foam rubber for comfort and cover with a washable fabric (Percey Hedley School, Newcastle).

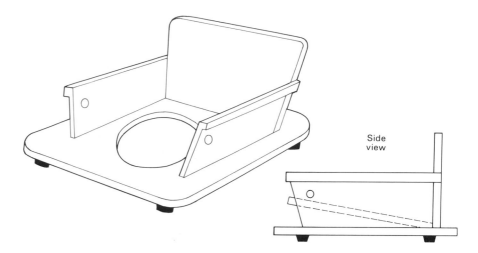

Side
view

Fig. 6.118 Toilet seat. Four rubber discs are fitted under the base to hold the seat in position. An angled seat may be added if necessary (Cheyne Spastic Centre, London).

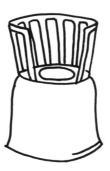

Fig. 6.119 Toilet seat.

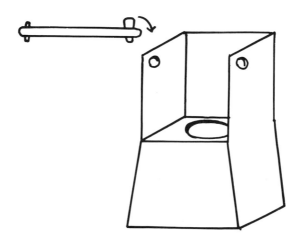

Fig. 6.120 Watford potty chair. The bar is made from 1 inch dowelling. For a tall child the back height needs increasing and the 10″ × 10″ seat needs enlarging. Feet must be flat on the floor. Use foot stool or box for increase of flexion of hips and knees for a very extended child.

STAGES IN THE DEVELOPMENT OF SITTING

0–3 MONTHS NORMAL DEVELOPMENTAL LEVEL

Common problems

Delay in lifting the head up if held fully supported in a sitting position, in holding the head steady. (Head lag in pull-to-sit, see Supine Development, p. 96.)

Abnormal performance of vertical head control. The head is held in an asymmetrical posture either laterally flexed, rotated or both. Arms, trunk and legs may be in infantile postures or other abnormal postures (see above).

Reflex reactions Extensor thrusts of head and trunk, the Moro reaction or occasionally asymmetrical tonic neck response both of which throw the child backwards and off balance. Flexor spasms may be present.

Treatment suggestions and daily care

Carry out any relevant methods suggested in Figs. 6.93 to 6.102, 6.106, but *giving support* to the child's shoulders and trunk and emphasising vertical head control.

3–6 MONTHS NORMAL DEVELOPMENTAL LEVEL

Common problems

Delay in sitting propped up in a chair with back and sides or similar support, in the straightening of the back from the dorsal area and subsequently of the whole back, sitting leaning on his hands for support. (Delay in overcoming head lag in pull-to-sit, see Supine Development, p. 96.)

Abnormal performance Anticipate 'Abnormal postures in sitting' above, which *may* be seen already in supported sitting. Support given to trunk only or shoulders only and by 6 months to waist and hips only.

Reflex reactions
1 Abnormal presence of abnormal extensor thrusts, flexion spasms, Moro or asymmetrical tonic neck reaction from 0–3 months.
2 Expect saving reactions forward only, if tipped in sitting.
3 Upright suspension of child and tilted sideways normally results in tilt or righting reaction but not yet in sitting positions (6 months).

Treatment suggestions and daily care

1   Carry out any relevant methods in Figs. 6.93 to 6.107, but decrease the amount of support so that trunk control can now develop.

2   Tip child whilst carrying him on your hip. Encourage him to come up to the vertical position again.

6–9 MONTHS NORMAL DEVELOPMENTAL LEVEL

Common problems

Delay in acquiring independent momentary sitting, sitting lean on one hand and use the other, inability to use a variety of sitting positions.

Abnormal performance
1   See 'Abnormal postures in sitting', above only *without* support to the child.
2   See Abnormalities of arm reach in Hand Function, p. 170.

Reflex reactions
1   Reactions 0–6 months developmental level may persist abnormally.
2   Expect saving reactions in the arms when falling sideways and forwards.
3   Expect head and trunk adjustment toward the vertical if the child is tipped *slowly* sideways, forward or backward.

Treatment suggestions and daily care

1   Carry out any relevant methods in Figs. 6.93–6.107 *without support* at this level of development.
2   Using methods for sitting whilst encouraging the child *to use one arm* movement whilst the other arm is grasping a support, leaning on a support or propping as a support. One arm is used for movements in feeding, dressing and playing (Chapter 7). Reaching down and in front with maintenance of sitting is only possible at this level.
3   Using methods for sitting with the child using *one leg movement*, such as stretching one leg up in the air to receive a shoe or sock, kick a ball or place foot on the seat of a chair. Sitting balance must be maintained without any back support, but *with* the child's own hand support (Figs. 6.121–6.123).

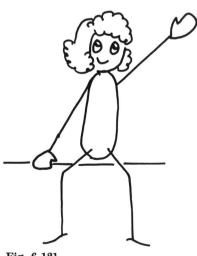

Fig. 6.121

4 See Supine Development, rise to sitting. Therapist may use baby gymnastics for head trunk-rising, to sitting from supine on mother's lap; astride sitting tipped sideways and raise to sit [96].
5 Unilateral arm or leg patterns whilst sitting is maintained, carried out by therapist (Fig. 6.121).

9–12 MONTHS NORMAL DEVELOPMENTAL LEVEL

Common problems

Delay in acquiring sitting steadily (for about 10 minutes) without support, on the floor and on a normal chair, sitting and playing without loss of balance, sitting and turning without falling; changing from one sitting position to another or to lying, to crawling or pulling up to standing; rising to, and from sitting.

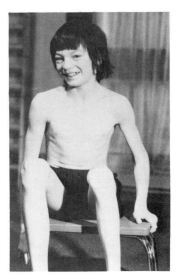

Fig. 6.122

Abnormal performance as described in 'Abnormal postures in sitting', but carried out *without* support. Abnormal patterns of rising to sitting, and changing positions.

Reflex reactions
1 Expect: positive tilt reactions sideways, forward and backward—saving reactions of the arms in all directions including backward.
2 Persistence of earlier reflex reactions as above.

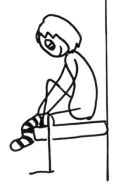

Fig. 6.123

Treatment suggestions and daily care

1 Use methods in Figs. 6.93 to 6.107) but with increased variety of arm patterns and no support of the child. Encourage his reaching overhead, across his body and behind his body. Use both arms simultaneously. Arm patterns selected should be those used to correct abnormal trunk postures e.g. the child's arm elevation corrects his kyphoscoliosis; his arm abduction and external rotation at his sides corrects round backs. (See Hand Function, p. 172.)

Changing postures into and out of sitting position or rising reactions
1 Rise into sitting from supine or prone (see Prone Development, Supine Development).
2 Rise from sitting to standing (see Standing Development, p. 163).
3 Sitting on the floor with legs in front of the child, change to prone.
   The child either places his hands in front of him, between his legs and goes down to lying, or he places one or both his hands to one side of him,

moves into side-sitting (Fig. 6.124) then down to lying. This pattern of changing to prone lying may also take place as a change to prone kneeling (crawling position) and back again (Fig. 6.125).

Fig. 6.124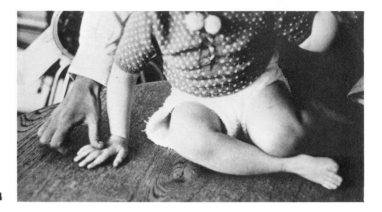

Fig. 6.125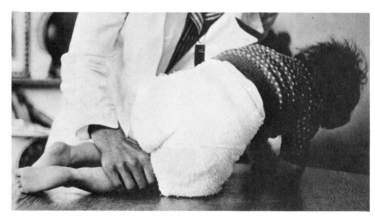

Training rolling (p. 98) emphasises rotation in the child's waist (body rotative reactions) and this pattern is used for these changes of position as well as for other rising reactions.

Many other changes of position from various sitting postures to lying or to kneeling or standing may have to be trained if they do not appear after a few basic changes of posture are taught to the child. Sometimes no normal pattern can be accomplished by the cerebral palsied child and his own patterns have to be observed and used (Figs. 6.71, 6.72).

The training of various rising reactions seen in normal children may often be corrective for any deformities in abnormal children. The movement involved activate postural fixation and counterpoising, although *transiently*, rotate the trunk, shoulder and pelvic girdles which result in relaxation of limb spasticity.

4   Train the child to get on and off low wide stools and then chairs (Fig. 6.126). He often has to use his hands as supports on the seat of the chair or

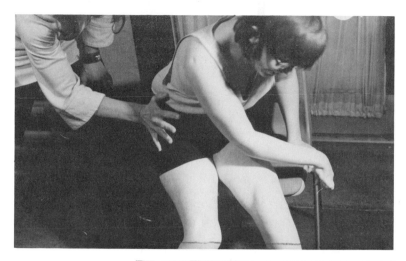

Fig. 6.126

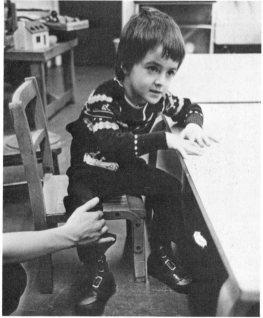

Fig. 6.127

grasp the back of the chair, the table nearby, or hook his arm over the chair or between the rungs of the chairback. Also train the child to get in and out of his wheelchair, in and out of a motor car, toy pedal car, tricycle and other apparatus.

Sitting on a chair and swivelling himself around on the chair is a useful motor ability which should also be trained (Fig. 6.127). Once again the postural change is corrective as it teaches separation of adducted legs, trunk control and arm extension from abnormal flexion of arms and back), as his hand reaches out for the back of the chair or therapist. Rising from sitting on a chair is now possible and this rising is discussed below (p. 163).

5   Practice a variety of sitting postures and reach and grasp in all directions in these postures. Sitting postures include side-sitting, (Fig. 6.124) sitting with one foot flat on the ground the other bent or straight, sitting with both knees bent and feet flat on the ground (crook-sitting), sitting in various types of chairs of the correct size and in adult chairs if the child is correctly placed.

6   Augment sitting with manual resistance given laterally, with rotation, anteroposteriorly (Fig. 6.107).

7   Tilt reactions and saving reactions in the limbs are stimulated by slow and by quick pushes (Fig. 6.128). Use rocking chairs, rocking horses, swings, see-saws rocker boat or toys, and inflatable toys to help develop the tilt reactions and security in sitting.

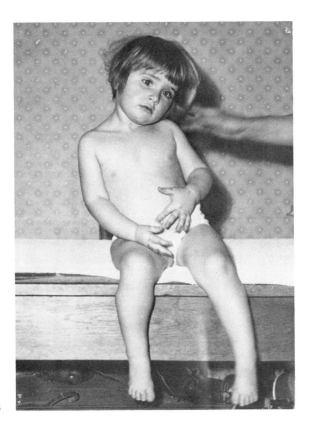

Fig. 6.128

DEVELOPMENT OF STANDING AND WALKING

The following main aspects should be developed:

Antigravity support or weight bearing on feet. Normally present at birth and modified at 6 months.

Postural fixation of the head on the trunk (Fig. 6.129) and on the pelvis in the vertical. Normally present by 9–12 months (see Sitting).

Postural fixation of the pelvic girdle in the vertical. Normally present by 9–12 months (see upright kneeling supported, and supported standing).

Counterpoising in the standing position when holding on (Fig. 6.130) i.e. normally at 9–12 months level, and without holding on, 12–18 months, becoming more varied in the 2nd and 3rd year of life. Examples are: lifting an arm or standing on one foot, holding on at 9–11 months normally and

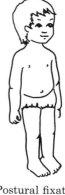

Fig. 6.129 Postural fixation, head on trunk on pelvis and whole of child in standing.

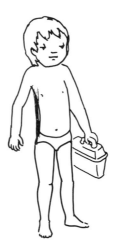

Fig. 6.130 Counterpoising a weight or movement of the arm.

much later, not holding on at 2½–3 years of age normally. Standing on one foot is a most important counterpoising reaction. The child can then take weight on one leg for long enough to allow the other to swing through and step.

Control of anteroposterior weight shift of the child's centre of gravity to initiate walking (propulsion) and to stop (retropulsion). Later in a diagonal direction and in turning (12–24 months normally).

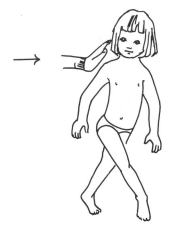

Fig. 6.131 Saving from falling with a protective step.

Control of lateral sway from one foot to the other. Normally developed in cruising and walking each hand held laterally, and similar activities about 12 months of age. Lateral sway is very obvious in toddlers and becomes modified with development.

Tilt reactions in standing are anteroposterior and lateral. They are acquired after standing and walking alone. Tilt reactions are not important for standing and walking. However children without tilt reactions will be unsure in the dark and on rough ground.

Saving from falling (Fig. 6.131) If tilt reactions fail the child will take a protective step out to save himself (staggering). He also flings out his arms in protective (saving) reactions. Normally these develop at 12–24 months of age. They are important as the child will have less fear of falling if he can protect himself, and may then become willing to walk.

Foley [81] has described various abnormalities of gait associated with the absence of one or more of the above mechanisms. These problems are treated in the practical suggestions below.

Rising reactions (6.132) from lying to standing (prone and supine) and from sitting to standing from kneeling to standing. Some have already been discussed in Supine, Sitting, Prone Development.

Note If a child cannot 'stand up', or rise and get up to standing, he may still *be able* to stand and walk. However he will depend on someone to place him in standing, and if this is not done standing and walking may be retarded for this reason.

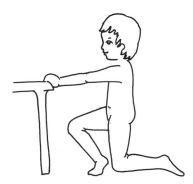

Fig. 6.132 Rising to standing.

STAGES IN DEVELOPMENT OF STANDING AND WALKING (Figs. 6.133–6.144)

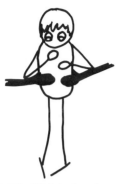

Fig. 6.133 Weight bearing on legs (supporting reaction) (*0–3 months*).

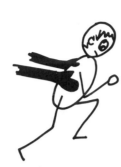

Fig. 6.134 Automatic stepping if infant is tilted forward (*0–3 months*).

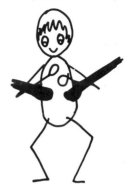

Fig. 6.135 Sinking or astasia (*3–6 months*).

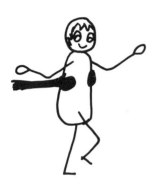

Fig. 6.136 Trunk supported standing and bouncing in standing (*5–7 months*).

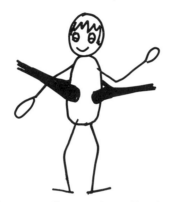

Fig. 6.137 Supported standing (*5–7 months*).

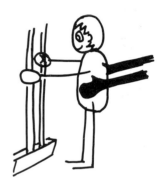

Fig. 6.138 Stand holding onto support with pelvic support (*7–9 months*).

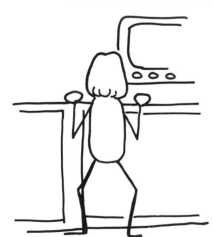

Fig. 6.139 Stand hold onto furniture (*7–9 months*).

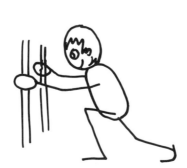

Fig. 6.140 Pull up to standing from various positions (*9–12 months*).

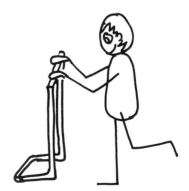

Fig. 6.141 Stand holding and lift one leg off the ground (*11 months*).

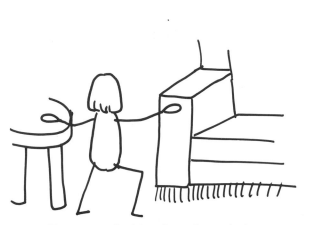

Fig. 6.142 Cruising (lateral stepping) (*9–12 months*).

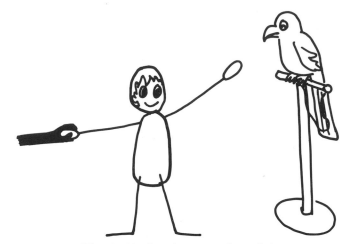

Fig. 6.143 Stand supported, reach in all directions (*9–12* months).

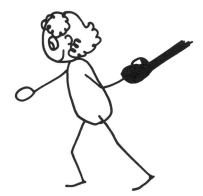

Fig. 6.144 Stand alone and walk with two, then one, then no hand support (*12–18 months*).

ABNORMAL POSTURES IN STANDING (see also Figs. 160, 164, 165).

These may be due to:

Absence of postural fixation The child may be able to maintain equilibrium, even inadequately, by attempting an abnormal posture to compensate for this absence (Fig. 6.145). He may be:

1 'Sinking' into hip flexion, knee flexion, with or without.
2 Adduction-internal rotation of the legs.
3 Lordosis may compensate for hip flexion.
4 Round back and head flexion may be present.
5 Feet in valgus or in overdorsiflexion. If overdorsiflexion is limited by tightness of ankle or plantarflexors, the child may stand on his toes.
    Alternatively the child may fall or extend backwards and compensate by (Figs. 6.146, 6.147):
1 Hip flexion.
2 Hyperextension of knees.
3 Internal rotation of legs, occasionally.
4 Valgus feet or normal feet.
5 Rounding his back and jutting his head forward.
    These postures, to maintain equilibrium under difficult circumstances, are also seen in normal people on slippery surfaces or when first attempting ice skating or skiing.

If the child also has spasticity or rigidity he may use that to prop himself up (see below). Spastic muscles shorten and maintain the abnormal postures above. They may create the abnormal postures in some children.

If the child has 'good' upper limbs or at least a grasp in poor upper limbs, he will use them for support. Such children 'stand and walk on their hands' with walking aids (Fig. 6.148). They bear so much weight on their hands that fatigue of the 'good' arms is common. Athetoids are known to hold their shoulders and arms forward and together to stop the backward fall.

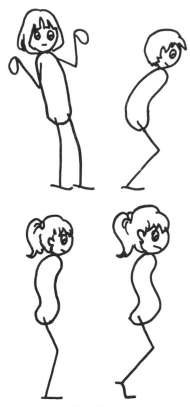

Fig. 6.145

Asymmetrical postural fixation and counterpoising The child will take weight on the better side and the leg with poor postural fixation will flex, adduct, internally rotate at the hip, flex at the knee and remain propped on the forefoot, or have no weight bearing. An athetoid may have one leg 'pawing' the ground with an involuntary motion.

Scoliosis may compensate for the body weight being distributed to one side only. This asymmetry may or may not also have been seen in other weight bearing positions such as sitting, kneeling or four foot kneeling. Sometimes, it is the postural fixation mechanism of the pelvis in standing only which fails, but which may be able to cope at lower levels of development.

The unaffected side in a hemiplegic obviously takes all or most of the child's weight. The hemiplegic leg is usually rotated back from the pelvis.

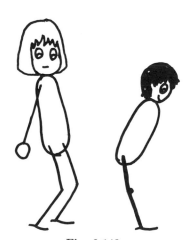

Fig. 6.146

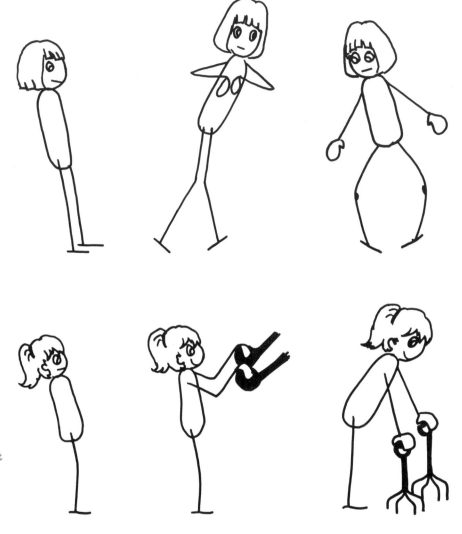

Fig. 6.147 Motor delay of standing. Compensation for lack of postural fixation (and thus falling backwards) by flexion-adduction of the hips and knees and pronation of feet, wide base, or by: hyperextension-abduction-internal rotation of knees, wide base, pronated feet.

Fig. 6.148 Compensation for lack of postural fixation and/or counterpoising in standing and/or standing on one foot by use of hand grasp or *walk on hands* for support. Spastic children increase spasticity in their arms if they flex and grasp.

It may be abducted or adducted, internally rotated, knee flexed, normal or hyperextended, and foot flat or in equinus, toes may claw the ground. If the young child's weight is taken on the hemiplegic leg and the good leg lifted, he may collapse or sink into flexion. Lack of counterpoise of one arm may lead to the child leaning abnormally to one side or onto the other hand for support. This creates asymmetrical postures. Presence of tilt reactions to *one* side only may be associated with scoliosis (Levitt [102]).

Absence of protective saving reactions of arms or legs may delay standing and walking in some children because of a justified fear of falling. This absence of saving will create crouching postures as seen in normal people who fear falling. In addition, absent tilt reactions make them even more unsure and they will increase those abnormal postures which occur to compensate for lack of postural fixation and counterpoising (Figs 6.145– 6.147). This is particularly obvious when they are on uneven surfaces.

Persistence of primitive reflexes and pathological reflexes   Unwitting constant stimulation of reflex stepping, excessive positive supporting reaction, 'lift reaction' [36], withdrawal reflexes increase abnormal leg postures (see p. 142). Repeated stimulation of one pattern of involuntary movement may increase tension in joint and abnormal posture may be seen. Persistence of abnormal reflexes on one side may be associated with abnormal supported standing postures e.g. Galant's reflex on one side of the trunk, asymmetrical tonic neck reflex to one side only and the everted withdrawal reflex or involuntary motion in one leg in an athetoid.

Growth of legs   Unequal growth of legs may be causing abnormal postures during standing e.g. weight bearing on the longer side leads to an equinus on the shorter leg in order to reach the ground. Weight bearing onto the shorter side leads to the hip flexing or both hip and knee flexing on the longer side to tend to equalise the balance. Scoliosis to one side may occur to compensate for leg length.

Asymmetrical distribution of spasticity may be present and add to the abnormal asymmetry in postural fixation or weight bearing in standing (see below).

Use of spasticity for compensation   If there are no postural fixation and counterpoising mechanisms and the child is spastic, he will *use his spasticity* to 'fix' him in the upright position. Thus if a child is 'standing on spasm' he will collapse to the ground if his spasticity is removed by physiotherapy or orthopaedic surgery to spastic muscle groups. He may be left with straight legs but completely loses his independent standing or even stumbling around.

Some athetoids have been observed to use an asymmetrical tonic neck reaction. The face turn to one side increases hypertonus in the weight bearing leg on that side, so that they can then bear weight on it.

It is interesting that some workers call spastics 'children with too much fixation' (Scrutton, [91]) and rigids 'children with too much postural stability' (Goff [56]). It is that they have *no* or poor normal postural fixation or stability and use hypertonicity to prop them up against gravity.

Biomechanics and spasticity   Spasticity may be greater in one group than other. If a resulting deformity is greater in one joint it leads to abnormal postures in the others to maintain a fairly upright position. These postures may also become deformities. For example:
1   Hip flexion may be dictated by greater knee flexion.

2 Hip flexion may be dictated by equinus in order not to extend 'on toes' and fall back.

3 Knee flexion may be dictated by too much hip flexion to avoid falling forward.

4 Hip flexion-adduction-internal rotation may be dictated by valgus flexed knees.

5 Hip extension may occur by hamstrings flexing the knees and tilting the pelvis backwards. A long kyphosis or a flat back may be associated.

6 Knee flexion or knee hyperextension may compensate for tight plantar-flexors or equinus.

7 Equinus may be secondary to excessive hip and knee flexion and the spastic plantarflexors cannot remain stretched by the mechanical over-dorsiflexion.

8 Lordosis compensates for hip flexion.

9 Kypholordosis compensates for hip flexion.

Clearly abnormal postures or deformities are rarely localised in one joint. Thus one spastic muscle group with its weak antagonists should never be considered alone in treatment, with or without orthopaedic surgery.

The spastic child's abnormal posture may be different when he has to maintain his balance on his own. Thus abnormal postures are:

Supported standing
Hip extension or semiflexion, adduction with legs together or crossing (scissoring), internal rotation.
Knee extension.
Equinus or 'on toes'.

Later in unsupported standing
Hip flexion, adduction-internal rotation.
Knee flexion or hyperextension or normal.
Feet equinovarus, varus (supination), valgus (pronation), sometimes heel may be down and forefoot everted.
Toes may clench and evert.
Lordosis, kyphosis, flattening of lumbar area or kypholordosis.
Pelvic tilt backwards is associated with flat back, pelvic tilt forwards with lordosis.

Arm and head postures

These are similar to the abnormal postures seen in the lower levels of the child's development. However, if the hands are grasped by an adult, or the child holds on for support he may use an abnormal pattern in arms and hands. The spastic child usually increases flexion-adduction in shoulder, shoulder hunching, flexion-pronation in elbow, palmar flexion with or without ulnar deviation in hands, adduction of thumbs. Increase in flexion in the arms often seems to increase flexion in the legs and aggravate the abnormal postures of the whole child, and vice versa. Increase of abnormal shoulder extension often associates with hip extension. Athetoids who abduct and hold their arms up abnormally with elbows flexed, also tend to grasp supports abnormally and aggravate their backward fall or lean. The child may flex his head or 'poke' his chin forward in standing.

ABNORMAL GAIT

The problems in standing will affect the gait, therefore walking should not be 'pushed' if standing is absent or very abnormal.

Delay or abnormal walking patterns may be due to:

Poor or absent postural fixation and counterpoising or asymmetrical ability to counterpoise   The child may 'waddle' from side to side without counterpoising each leg, that is he 'falls' from foot to foot as he cannot maintain posture for any length of time on one side. There may be excessive trunk sway from side to side. The pelvis and trunk may rotate forward on the side of the 'swing-through' (*stepping*) leg instead of counterpoising on to the weight bearing leg in an upright position. The child may have a better postural mechanism on one side, most obviously seen in hemiplegia or asymmetrical quadriplegias or triplegias (asymmetrical ability). A limp onto the good side is then characteristic of the gait.

Athetoids may 'run headlong' as they cannot bear weight long enough on each side for a step. Athetoids and ataxics stumble about for this and other reasons. Cerebral palsied children, mentally subnormal children and others who are only motor delayed, will not wish to walk, show fear of walking and hang on to adults excessively and onto their walking aids. Excessive arm flinging movements or emphasis of the saving reactions in the arms come into play to help the child balance on each unstable leg. 'Sinking' patterns of standing and compensation for falling back are seen as in Standing (see Figs. 6.145 to 6.148).

Absence of anteroposterior shift   This makes it impossible for the child to *start* walking. A walking aid on wheels may start him off. Stopping is also difficult if this mechanism is not operating. He may also 'mark time' and then stop, as he is unable to stop or reverse the anteroposterior shift. Some children only stop by collapse onto their bottoms.

Absence of lateral sway   This is obvious in the athetoid 'running headlong' and other children pushing wheelwalkers. In treatment, this is closely allied with training standing on one foot (counterpoising), and is developed in cruising sideways and other activities.

Lack of tilt reactions in prone, supine, sitting, upright kneel and standing rarely delays walking. This training in walking should not be delayed if these reactions are not yet acquired. Purdon-Martin found that labyrinthectomised adults could walk although tilt reactions were not possible without their labyrinths [30]. Similar observations have been noted in children who walk but have absent or poor tilt reactions. Nevertheless tilt reactions should be included in the programme as it makes the child more steady in changes of terrain and in the dark. As Dr. Foley puts it 'you cannot walk across a ploughed field at night if you do not have tilt reactions' [81].

Saving or Protective Reactions (*arms and legs*)   These must be trained to prevent the danger of the child falling on his face, and giving him confidence to walk. Remember that the protective step in falling is not the same as a voluntary step which the child takes as he is being trained to walk. Foley [81] observed the presence of voluntary stepping without the presence of protective stepping and vice-versa. Therapy must therefore train both of those stepping movements. Excessive saving reactions in arms or legs may occur to compensate for the absence of the other mechanisms. It is most noticeable in ataxics and athetoids. The 'drunken walk' may be excessive staggering reactions in the legs. Athetoids cannot 'stand still' but take little protective steps.

Spastic gaits

All the problems above will be included with the addition of the pull of spasticity and associated weakness. There may be abnormal postures which are associated with each other, as described in Standing (p. 142).

Hips and knees

Hips may adduct and cross when the child is supported, and adduct-internally rotate and flex when the child is walking independently. Flexion occurs as the leg is swinging through and/or on weight bearing (stance).

Knees may overflex on swing through and on weight bearing. Hip and knee flexion may occur to allow a plantarflexed foot (or toe pointing foot) to swing and clear the ground, and once on the ground hip and knee flexion occur to push the heel to the ground. 'Toe first' and not the normal heel strike is common in spastics.

Lack of heel strike after 'swing through' may be compensated differently.

In hemiplegia and other spastics the hip alone may flex with hyperextension of the knee to press the heel to the ground. This is usual with 'extensor spasticity' or excessive antigravity support as the forefoot strikes the ground.

A wide base is used with flexed adducted (valgus) knees as the spastic child cannot balance on the small base created by adduction of the hips.

Feet

Walking on the toes is seen if the child is supported and later when he walks alone. There is not only weight bearing on the toes but the toes are brought down first for weight bearing (see above).

Walking on the toes may become walking on a pronated-everted (valgus) foot in the child's efforts to compensate for spastic plantarflexors.

Walking on toes may be accompanied by slightly flexed hips and even straight knees or slightly flexed in younger or milder cases.

A rare *normal* 'ballerina walk' has been observed (Holt [105]). Hips and knees are straight and flexible.

Pelvis and trunk

The pelvis often rotates abnormally in spastic gaits. The rotation may be backwards so the leg appears 'retracted' and behind the other. Usually the front, better leg may take more weight, as in hemiplegia. However the 'back leg' may take more weight and allow the forward leg to step, take its momentary weight and then transfer onto the back leg, which only has time to take a small step and *cannot* get in front of the forward leg.

Pelvic tilt is also backwards with flattening of the lumbar area, or pelvic tilt forwards with a lordosis of the lumbar area. Kyphosis of the thorax may occur with flat back or lordosis. Scoliosis may be present due to unequal weight distribution, leg length and other reasons.

If the child takes a step, his spasticity may be so great that he has to lean back to push his leg forward. He has an anteroposterior 'waddle' or jerky walk. Lateral waddle is associated with spastic adductors and weak abductors. It is also involved with inability to fixate the pelvis when counterpoising in standing on one leg. The trunk and head may lean forward to help overcome spasticity as well as maintain balance (see above). This usually *increases* toe walking as the child cannot put his heels down in this pattern.

Arms

Excessive arm swing up, held in the air, or excessive saving reactions may occur in the arms. Therefore, normal reciprocal arm swing may be absent. Abnormal postures of arms may be seen as in earlier motor developmental skills. The retraction of the shoulder may accompany retraction of the pelvis and hip. See Figs. 6.160–6.167.

Summary

Abnormal features of gait for therapy

Excessive **1** Hip and trunk sway from side to side or a pelvic 'waddle'.

2   Hip and trunk sway anteroposterior and jerky gait.

3   Asymmetry of weight bearing and unequal steps.

4   Abnormal postures of head, trunk, pelvis, knees and feet.

5   Abnormal stepping patterns, e.g. walk on toes.

6   Athetoid 'running gait'; 'drunken gait' of ataxics or athetoids; 'high stepping gait' or 'scissoring gait' in spastics or
athetoids.

7   Overactive arms to maintain balance, 'tight rope walking' or
abnormal arm postures and lack of reciprocal arm swing.

TREATMENT SUGGESTIONS AT ALL LEVELS OF DEVELOPMENT

Practical points

Train standing (fixation and counterpoising) and postural alignment *first*,
and also when child is walking independently, but with an abnormal gait.
All the abnormal gaits discussed above will be treated in a programme
concentrating on:

1   Equal distribution of weight on each foot.

2   Correction of abnormal postures.

3   Building up of the child's stability by decreasing support.

4   Delay training in standing and walking if the child is not ready.

5   Continuing to develop head, trunk and pelvic postural fixation and
counterpoising in sitting, on hands and knees, half-kneeling and positions
other than standing, as well as in standing.

6   Weight shift leading to stepping.

7   Training lateral sway and cruising and walk holding support each side.

8   Training stopping and starting and turning and walking on uneven
ground, and using stairs and inclines.

1   Equal distribution of weight bearing on each foot   Supported and later unsupported standing

1   Check this by having child standing on two weighing scales and help
him correct this as you read the *equal* weight borne on each scale.

2   Head and trunk in midline supported and then unsupported after 9
month level of normal development.

3   Teach weight shift onto the side that bears less weight. Do this by
asking and assisting the child to move himself onto the leg. If possible, ask
the child to move against your hand placed firmly against his lateral hip.

4   Use a mirror for both you and the child to see that he is in correct
alignment with his weight on both feet.

5   Use a wide base and then bring both feet together for standing, then
move one foot in front of the other.

6 Correct any deformities, especially of the feet, such as equinus, so that there are *two* plantigrade feet for equal weight bearing. Equinus may be secondary to other deformities, see below.

7 Check length of legs in case of growth asymmetries and raise shoe if there is more than $\frac{1}{2}$-inch difference.

8 Remember to keep the child's weight forward over both feet and not allow him to twist or lean backwards. Do *not* let him *lean back* against the wall, standing apparatus or an adult.

2 Correct abnormal postures or deformities See correction of abnormal postures in sitting and use the same methods for kyphosis, scoliosis, hip adduction and internal rotation, feet deformities.

1 Place the child's legs apart in standing, hips and knees turned outward with head and back upright, knees straight and feet flat on the ground, facing outwards. Stand him like this over a roll of blankets, inflatable toy, sponge rubber, large stuffed toy or wide toy truck. You can hold him like this when you are seated on the floor and the child's legs are abducted over your thigh or legs. Hold the child's knees and thighs facing apart and outward (in external rotation). The toy he straddles may have to keep his *knees and feet* apart. Press his heels to the ground by pushing down through his knees to his heels.

2 Equal weight distribution and weight forward over feet will correct many abnormal postures. Symmetrical postures and head in midline corrects asymmetry. Motivate and facilitate child's arm reach overhead to overcome a rounded back or bent hips and knees (Fig. 6.105).

3 In all methods the arms should be either in symmetrical extension at his sides; or at right angles at his shoulders, over a roll or on a couch; or with the weight of the child taken through his elbows or through his hands; or with the child grasping a bar in front of him with his *elbows extended* or bars at each side of him, or broomsticks, with elbows extended. The child should keep his head in the centre and his back as straight as possible (Fig. 6.149).

4 Splints and braces. If abnormal positions cannot be actively corrected by the child *in every joint*, at the same time, splintage or bracing should be used for one joint whilst the others are actively corrected by him. For example, correct abnormal adduction with abduction pants or an abduction splint, whilst training the child to stretch his knees and keep his heels down with his weight taken towards the external surface of his feet. Another possibility is to correct bent knees with the knee corsets, or polythene knee pieces, whilst the child actively corrects the position of hips and feet. Yet another possibility is to correct the feet in below-knee irons or in plaster-of-Paris whilst the child actively corrects hips and knees, head and trunk.

Orthopaedic surgery in selected cases having hip flexion-adduction-internal rotation, knee flexion and equinus, equinovarus or equinovalgus and postoperative physiotherapy (see Chapter 8) [83, 84].

3 Building up child's own stability by a decrease of support given to him

Carry out methods with trunk or shoulders supported by your hands, standing frame or standing box. Then hold the child supported at his waist, then hips, then thighs and knees. This is equivalent to developmental levels 0–9 months. At 9–11 months his own hand grasp is spontaneously used for support, but before this, the child's hands will have to be placed onto bars for grasp.

Note Weight bearing and stepping are not walking Children who are able to bear weight and reflex step without trunk balance are really at 0–6 months normal developmental level. These children are frequently the ones who support themselves under their arms in walking frames on wheels and run headlong in them. Some athetoids who run headlong, but are unable to stand alone, are mostly at this developmental level, having not yet developed the postural fixation of head, trunk and pelvis of later trimesters. Some ataxics can also bear weight and step in walkers. If there are wheels on the walkers, they will stagger in all directions. The training of standing and walking in such children, including athetoids and ataxics, should concentrate on the next trimesters of development which build up trunk and pelvic control.

4 Delay the training of standing and walking in the following instances:

1 Abnormal weight bearing, without the trunk and pelvic control of later (3–9 months) levels of development, may be particularly severe. If excessive antigravity reaction of hip adduction ('scissoring') internal rotation, hip and knee extension, toe standing occurs when the child is held in standing and this reaction cannot be corrected, or only corrected with difficulty, by the therapist, then the training of standing should be *delayed*. This is frequently a problem with spastics. Treatment in these cases should concentrate on prone, supine and sitting development.

2 Delay standing and walking in the case when the excessive antigravity reaction (supporting reaction) is only controlled at the cost of 'abnormal overflow'. The reaction can be controlled and corrected manually or by equipment, so that the legs are kept apart, knees straight facing out and heels down. However, the leg postures may be correct *but* at the cost of an increase of hypertonus in the arms and hands, or trunk. Check whether this 'overflow' can be corrected at once. If not, although the development of standing may proceed, there will be a loss or decrease of hand function or increase of deformity in the upper limbs and trunk. Thus, treatment suggestions for standing should be followed when the child is more ready to respond to them. This will be after a period of training the pelvic and trunk fixation mechanisms in prone, supine and sitting development and occasionally in upright kneeling. Development of these postural mechanisms does seem to decrease excessive hypertonus during weight bearing on the feet when these children are finally placed in standing.

5 Continue training of head, trunk and pelvic control in other developmental levels during training of standing. Train this control in sitting and on hands and knees, and upright kneeling, and emphasise postural fixation and counterpoising mechanisms. *Do not use upright kneeling* if the child has hip flexion-tightness or lordosis. Even if the older child is walking, these mechanisms may still have to be trained, to *improve* his pattern of walking (gait). See 0–12 months developmental levels below, for these mechanisms in standing development.

Points **6**, **7** and **8** above are discussed in the developmental level 9–12 months, below, as well as in later development.

STAGES IN THE DEVELOPMENT OF STANDING AND WALKING

0–3 MONTHS NORMAL DEVELOPMENTAL LEVEL

Common problems

Delay in taking weight on feet, when supported on soles.

Abnormal performance See 'Abnormal postures in standing' supported (p. 142), see reflex reactions (p. 141).

Reflex reactions
1 Excessive antigravity response, see Abnormal postures (p. 142).
2 Persistence of automatic stepping after 1–2 months.
3 Various abnormal stepping reactions such as 'athetoid dance', when each leg withdraws outwards with eversion on sole contact with the ground. Sole contact may also include 'grasping' reflex of the ground. Some athe- this 'conflict between grasp and withdrawal reflexes' (Twitchell [91]), in one leg only a 'pawing' repetitive involuntary motion of this leg.
4 Excessive 'crossed extension reflex' seen in a jerky high stepping pattern, with the other leg rigidly extended as its sole contacts the ground. This is similar to automatic stepping above.
5 Withdrawal reflex of both feet on contact with the ground, as opposed to alternate withdrawals of each leg.

Treatment suggestions and daily care

Increase weight bearing on both feet which counteracts delay as well as the various abnormal reactions to foot contact with floor.

1 Use of knee corsets, polythene knee-pieces, long leg irons or braces (Appendix).
2 Periods of weight bearing in apparatus e.g. frames, standing boxes or cut out tables (Fig. 6.149). (Appendix.)
3 Joint compression through hips and pelvis or through knees (Fig. 6.150).
4 Desensitise soles of feet by weight bearing on feet with heels pressed down in sitting, squatting and in standing. Use shoes and various floor surfaces, sponge or a trampoline etc. to find which the child can tolerate.

Correct abnormal postures within methods in Fig. 6.149.

Note   Give full trunk support for use of methods at this level (Fig. 6.149).

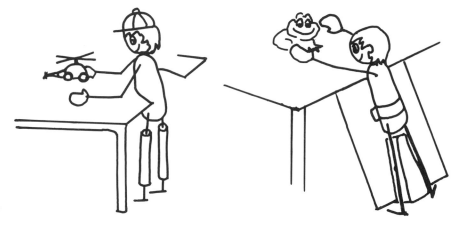

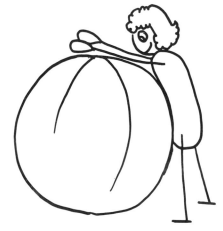

Fig. 6.149 Child's arms symmetrical, head and trunk central, weight equal on each foot. Keep child's weight forward onto his feet. Trunk is supported by a roll, a large ball, table, high couch or the body of the therapist behind him. Also use a high couch, ledges on an ordinary table with padded edge, rounded edge or cut-out table. Later remove the trunk support and use his hand grasp on support, or lean only on forearms, lean on hands on low table (9–12 months level) and then higher tables. Legs are apart and externally rotated, hips flexed or extended, knees straight, feet flat on the ground. Use apparatus or abduction pants, knee corsets, foot supports according to the child's difficulties. To assume corrected position use methods in Figs. 6.168–6.172.
Rhythmically shift the knees into semi-flexion to avoid rigid infantile stance. Hold his knees to do this, especially if the knees also hyperextend. Later shift weight from foot to foot (see Fig. 6.152).

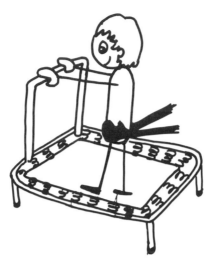

Fig. 6.150 Joint compression through hips, later through knees. Child may stand on floor, but trampoline, sponge rubber, inflatable mattress may be used if posture is kept corrected, and *bouncing is restricted*. The trunk may be supported by his own grasp or holding your shoulders (9–12 months level) or if his trunk requires more support (6–9 months level) lean child against table, roll, couch, large stuffed stable toy, or large ball. Head and body alignment must be well over straight legs and feet on the ground. Avoid hyperextension of knees and any abnormal postures as in Figs. 6.145–6.148, p. 139

3–5 MONTHS NORMAL DEVELOPMENTAL LEVEL

This is the level at which the normal baby does not take weight in standing but sags (astasia). The next level of development should be attempted from time to time until there is a flicker of response, then work at 6–9 months level on the development of standing.

6–9 MONTHS NORMAL DEVELOPMENTAL LEVEL

Common problems

Delay in weight bearing with flexible knees, if supported, active 'bounce' when held in standing, alternate stepping (not automatic high stepping), if held with hip flexion, knee extension and heels down on the floor and beginning to stand alone grasping a support.

Abnormal performance   See 'Abnormal posture in standing', supported, above.

Reflex reactions   Those expected to develop at this level are:
1   Parachute or saving reactions in the arms on falling forward or sideways (see Sitting, p. 113).
2   Propping reactions in the arms to 'break' the fall (see Sitting, p. 112).
3   Tilt reactions in sitting which may make standing more secure if not directly related to its acquisition.
4   Presence of toe clenching in supported standing until about 9 months

level.

5 Persistence of reflex reactions from 0–3 months is abnormal.

9–12 MONTHS NORMAL DEVELOPMENTAL LEVEL

Common problems

Delay in standing, holding on and releasing one hand, releasing one leg to stand on the other, stepping sideways or cruising. Inability to stand alone momentarily, step two-handed support, one-handed support. Delay in rise from prone or supine to standing with help given in the transitional positions of either sitting, kneeling on all fours and half-kneeling. Delay in pulling himself to standing from kneeling holding on, from sitting or from hands and knees.

Abnormal performance of standing posture, see 'Abnormal posture in standing', supported and unsupported (above), 'Abnormal Gait', above.

Reflex reactions   Those expected at this level are the saving reactions in the arms if falling backwards as well as others already present (see sitting development, p. 112).

Physiotherapy suggestions

See Figs. 6.149 and 6.150 but remove support from child's trunk, and later from pelvis.

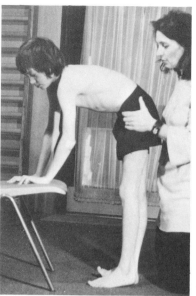

Fig. 6.151

Improve stability with the following techniques: the child stands, holding on or alone. Apply manual pressure at his hips or shoulders pushing him off balance, he must actively maintain his upright standing—'Don't let me push you over'. Do this laterally and also anteroposteriorly (Fig. 6.151). Do this with rotation—'Don't let me turn you'. Another way of using resistance is to ask the child to push against your hands placed in positions on his hips or shoulders or on one hip and one shoulder—'Push against my hands'. Resistance should not be *so great* that the child twists his limbs into abnormal positions, or increases involuntary movements, or even falls over!

Stand and sway (Figs. 6.151–6.153)   Train lateral sway with legs apart then together. At first the child is swayed from side to side, then shifts his weight along or against your hand on his hip, shoulder, or hip and shoulder. Augment weight shift against your hand offering resistance. Carry this out initially with support to trunk or child on forearms, on hands, or grasping a support with elbows straight.

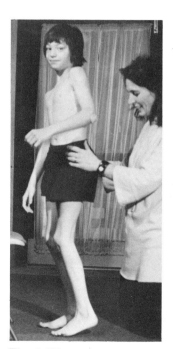

Fig. 6.152

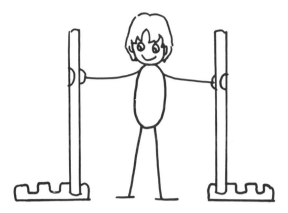

Fig. 6.153

Child's grasp should be forward, sideways at waist and at shoulder level. Lateral grasp on poles is preferable to parallel bars as it improves symmetrical weight bearing, back and head position and trains supinated grasp. Release grasp as soon as control is possible without it. Lateral sway prepares child for cruising and is part of good gait training.

Sway child *forward and back* (anteroposterior shift) (Figs. 6.154 and 6.155). Child shifts his weight forward and back. Child shifts his weight against your hands placed first on anterior-superior iliac crests or on his gluteii. Weight shift forward initiates stepping.

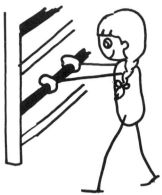

Fig. 6.154

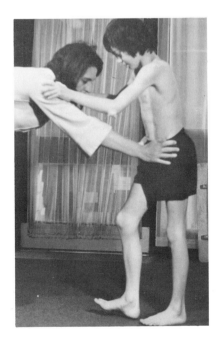

Fig. 6.155

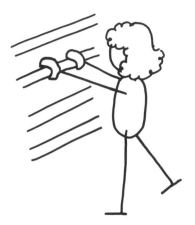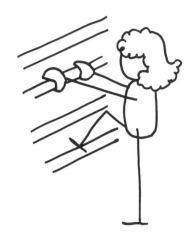

Fig. 6.156

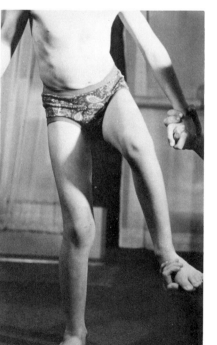

Fig. 6.157

Standing and counterpoising (Figs. 6.156 and 6.157) The child stands holding on with both hands, then one hand, whilst lifting one leg to different heights on the bar or in the air. He should lift one of his legs up in front, to the side and backward, on to bars, box step, a beachball, onto your hand, or to have his shoe put on or off. He should also stand and reach in all directions for toys offered to him, and stand supported, bend down and come up. He should also walk hands down the bars, and fetch a toy hung on the bottom bar or on a high bar.

Train standing and counterpoising using the facilitation of arm and leg patterns The child stands grasping support; hold his weight bearing leg in external rotation, while he moves the other leg using various patterns. Facilitate the patterns against resistance by holding correctly as *must be shown clinically* (p. 155).

Leg patterns that may be used are flexion-adduction external rotation (stepping pattern) from and to extension-abduction-internal rotation (push-off pattern), the knee extended and foot dorsiflexed in 'stepping'. Hold toes and forefoot in dorsiflexion in 'push-off' and to prevent extensor thrust. Arm patterns should also be used in the following ways. With the child standing holding a support with one hand or leaning on one hand correctly facilitate the other arm into elevation-abduction-external rotation against resistance or in assisted or active reaching for a toy overhead. He could also stand while 'walking' his hands up the wall or sliding up the wall or a soapy mirror or other play activities. Also facilitate all other arm patterns in standing (see p. 173).

Note Use leg and arm patterns *without* giving resistance if excessive overflow of spasticity cannot be controlled and if methods are not correctly carried out.

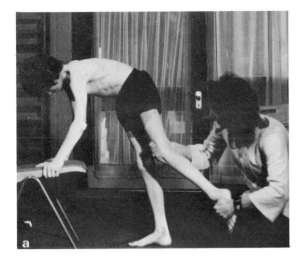 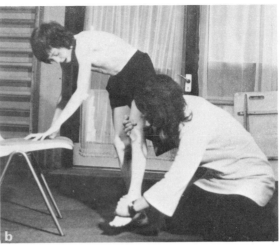

Fig. 6.158 Correction of stepping pattern, i.e. facilitation of leg flexion-external rotation, knee extension with dorsiflexion. 'Push-off' pattern, a. 'Heel strike' pattern, b.

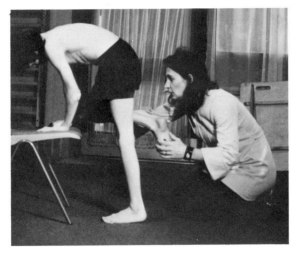

Fig. 6.159 From this hip-knee flexion-abduction-internal rotation pattern facilitate 'stance' of extension-adduction-external rotation.

Correction of abnormal postures The arm and leg patterns used are also used to correct abnormal positions of the arms and legs. In addition rotation of the pelvis and trunk with the arm or leg movements decreases hypertonus and improves postures (see Arm Patterns, p. 174).

Correction of some common abnormal postures in standing and walking These are from approximately the 9 month developmental level (supported) to over 12 month developmental level (unsupported).

Fig. 6.160 Correction of a flexed child whose limbs may also adduct and internally rotate, in standing or in walking. Keep child's weight forward as in these exercises, there is a tendency to lean too far backwards. Arms are extended and externally rotated. This corrects head, trunk and legs. Hold child's shoulders, elbows or grasp hands. Encourage weight shift from side to side by tipping child from your hold on his arms. Stand and walk by pushing walker at shoulder level. Open hands, pushing rather than pulling overcomes too much flexion. Keep elbows straight, elbow splints (gaiters) may be needed. Knee corsets to maintain extension of knees and/or to get heels down if required. Calipers may be needed in older children. Slow walk and a long lunge forward when stepping and pushing truck and therapist will stretch tight heelcords and tight knee flexors.

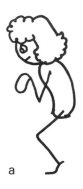

a

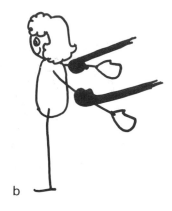

b

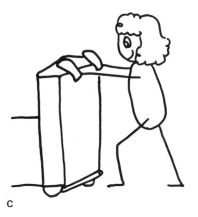

c

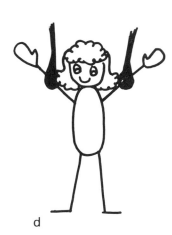

d

1 Flexion and 'sinking' posture (Fig. 6.160).
2 Asymmetrical posture (Fig. 6.161).
3 Internal rotation of legs (Fig. 6.162).
4 Hip extension, knee flexion, plantarflexion, arm flexion also for arm abduction-extension in the air, elbow flexion, wrist palmarflexion (arms in 'high guard') (Figs. 6.163 and 6.164).
5 Hyperextended knees and lordosis (Figs. 6.165 and 6.166).

Correction of a 'waddling gait' or 'running headlong' must include training of lateral sway and this is also developed in cruising around furniture. This 9–12 months level of development includes the important cruising.

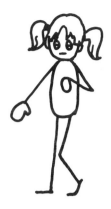

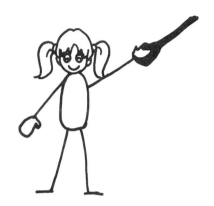

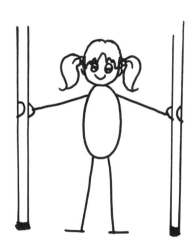

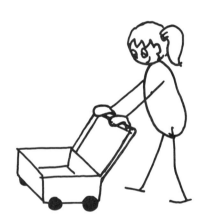

Fig. 6.161 Weight bearing on to more affected side or on to hemiplegic side. Hold arm in position to counteract arm flexion-adduction-internal rotation. Bring arm forward if shoulder retracts. Symmetrical grasp, or *both* hands open and pushing truck. Use elbow splints to maintain elbow extension. Weight distributed equally on feet. Shift weight to more affected side. Child should grasp with his arms apart and turned out or with his arms abducted in mid-position but *not* with shoulders turned inward.

Cruising or stepping sideways The child holds parallel bars and takes a step sideways. He should not step with hip flexion but with abduction only. At first hold, then ask him to keep his pelvis and/or trunk upright, so that he takes weight through his standing leg. Improve this activity by joint compression through the standing hip or knee whilst manual resistance is given to the abduction movement of the stepping leg. Some children respond to resistance without the joint compression through the weight bearing leg. Others may require you to correct any abnormal positions of hip, knee and foot by holding the thigh and knee extended and externally rotated, and the child's weight on the outside of the foot. In 'walk holding two hands' below use technique to train weight shift sideways which also helps cruising.

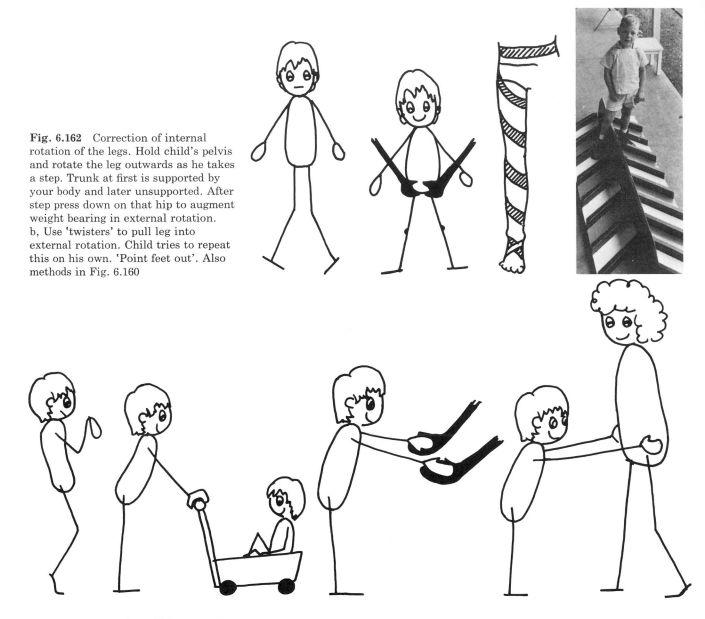

Fig. 6.162 Correction of internal rotation of the legs. Hold child's pelvis and rotate the leg outwards as he takes a step. Trunk at first is supported by your body and later unsupported. After step press down on that hip to augment weight bearing in external rotation.
b, Use 'twisters' to pull leg into external rotation. Child tries to repeat this on his own. 'Point feet out'. Also methods in Fig. 6.160

Fig. 6.163 Correction of hip extension, knee flexion, arm flexion, plantar flexion (toe walk). For arm abduction-extension in the air, elbow flexion, wrist palmar flexion.

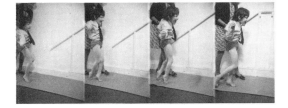

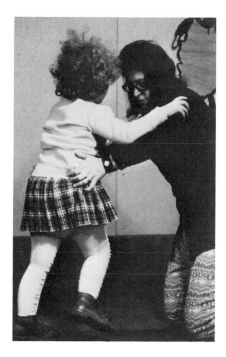

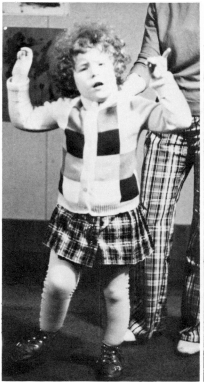

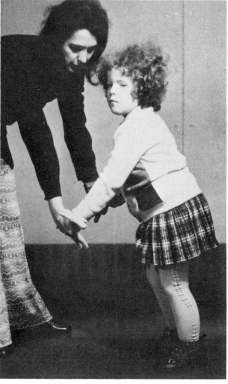

Fig. 6.164 Correction of hip extension, knee flexion, arm flexion, plantar flexion (toe walk). For arm abduction-extension in the air, elbow flexion, wrist palmar flexion.

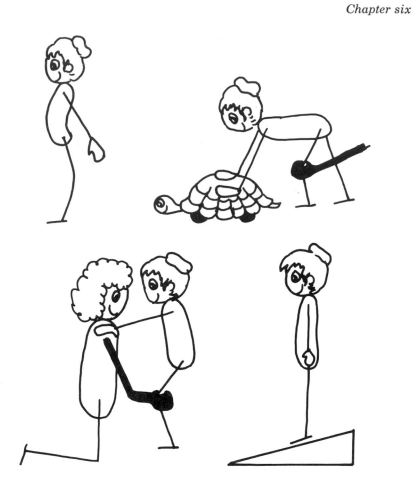

Fig. 6.165 Correction of hyperextended knees and lordosis.

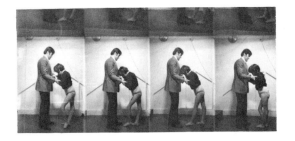

Fig. 6.166
Hyperextended knees and lordosis.

Walk holding two hands or one hand This developmental level of walking (normally about 12–13 months) is the level at which children are functioning when they walk with walking aids of many different types. The walkers stimulate locomotor reactions of initiation of stepping and lateral sway.

1 Walk holding parallel bars or parallel ropes. If the child has not yet achieved grasp and release, a felt cuff or moving hand grip which slides along the bar may be used.
2 Walk with a walking frame grasping in front or at the sides, e.g. Rollator or Amesbury.
3 Walking holding someone's hands on either side or in front of him.
4 Walk pushing a weighted doll's pram, another child in his wheelchair a child's chair, a kitchen chair, a chair on wooden skis or with set of runners, or a metal walker on four points which slide (Appendix).
5 Walking using crutches, elbow crutches, tripods, quadripods or sticks.
6 Walking using vertical poles at either side with thick rubber bases (Fig. 6.161)

When using walking aids consider the following:
Grasping a support at the side of the child tends to train lateral sway for walking. However, if the support involves elbow flexion this may be contra-indicated in spastics as the grasp-elbow flexion and hunching of the shoulders increases spasticity in the arms and may also overflow into the legs. The hand grasp should therefore be low and if necessary elbow splints used to keep the elbows extended (Fig. 6.167).

Grasping the hand support in front helps to train the anteroposterior shift needed to start walking. However, if the child bends his elbows with hand grasp this may throw his weight backward and disturb his development of standing balance. He should use straight elbows and lean on both his hands flat or forward onto his grasp. This is most effective in training the initiation of stepping and continuation of stepping. In Fig. 6.164, note the open hands of the therapist allowing the child to press down and forward to initiate stepping.

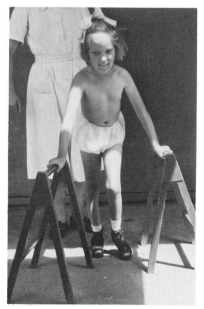

Incorporation of the hands whilst training walking in, say, some athetoids and ataxics or any children with servere perceptual problems interferes with the use of crutches or sticks, which become too difficult to manage. Fixed Padded Skis to chairs, stable walking frames, weighted trolleys and prams should be used instead. Later crutches with weighted bases may be managed by some children.

Fig. 6.167

Children who run headlong in walkers should have them weighted or a brake on the back wheel, or have wheels in front only or not at all. If the child sits on the rim of the walker or leans forward dragging his feet, the walker must be slowed down or weighted or wheels removed. Concentrate on standing balance in treatment care of these children.

Grasping with one hand is usually a progression from walking holding on with two hands. However, if the child takes weight abnormally through one side more than the other or if there are asymmetrical postures, then *two* aids should be used, until he walks alone. Some children progress to grasping one 'clumper' or stick in the centre and in front of them, instead of using two aids.

A child 'walking on his hands' and *'hanging on his armpits'* in walking aids so that he hardly takes weight on his feet should be discouraged from doing so. If not he will step in this way for years and his independent walking will not have any opportunity of developing. Give extra training in all aspects of head trunk and pelvic stability in both standing and sitting development for these children.

Abnormal postures of the head, trunk and legs should be corrected (Figs. 6.160–6.167). If correction is not possible with a particular walking aid then a better one should be found, or perhaps walking with aids not trained at all. In such cases rather train the earlier levels in the development of standing or walking more thoroughly.

Note Pushing a trolley with handles which are too low or sticks and clumpers which are too low may increase head and back rounding.

Walking aid giving too much aid Always assess the child's own ability to weight bear, step, control head and trunk and pelvis, and grasp before supporting him in these abilities.

Fig. 6.168 Assume standing from prone lying across a roll, large ball or bed. Check that heels are on the ground, knees, hips straight and if necessary, turned outward.

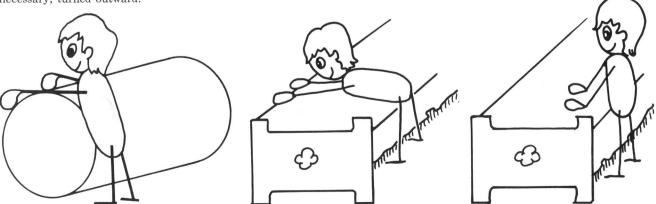

Rising to Standing (0–12 months)
Prone to Standing (Fig. 6.168) At earlier developmental levels the child
has learnt to roll over and get on to his hands and knees or rise from prone
onto hands and knees (0–6 months). Train him to rise to half-kneeling then
to standing (6–12 months) see Prone Development (p. 91).

Supine to standing Rising from supine to sitting into squatting on both
or one foot and pulling up to standing may be easier for the child. Help him
to develop this by taking both his hands when he is sitting on the ground.
Stabilise his foot with your foot and wait for him to pull himself forward
over his feet and then extend his legs. The full rising can be carried out
from supine to squatting and up to standing by holding the child's hands
and feet flat on the table. Hemiplegic or asymmetrical children can be
encouraged to take weight on the more affected side as they squat and rise
(see Supine Development, pp. 96 and 165).

Sitting to standing Rising from sitting on a chair (Fig. 6.169) or from
squatting to standing (Fig. 6.170) can be carried out with manual resistance
applied on the top of the child's thighs. The child's thighs should be kept
apart and in external rotation by the therapist who is either behind or in
front of the child. If the therapist sits on the ground in front of the child
she has the advantage of making sure that his weight comes forward and
well over his feet. Getting the child's 'nose over his toes' is important or he
will not become independent in rising. He will tend to use an extensor
thrust or get up abnormally by pushing on his feet, leaning backwards
and grasping your hands, being totally dependent on you in order to rise
to his feet. He may learn to bring his own weight forward over his feet if
he is also told to reach forward and down to the floor and *raise his bottom*
off the chair. In some children resistance may be given at the lumbar area

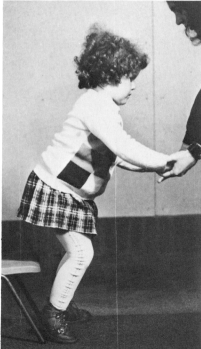

Fig. 6.169

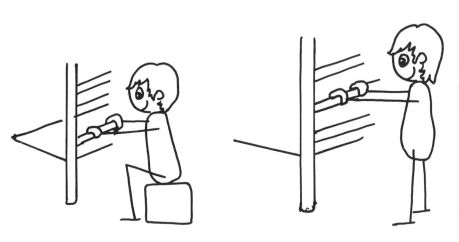

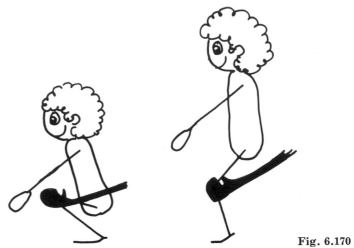

Fig. 6.170

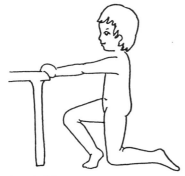

Fig. 6.171

to augment this movement. Rising from the floor and from a chair to standing must be taught by careful verbal instruction. For example rising from a chair involves—'Put your feet flat on the ground, bring your nose over your toes, lift your bottom, stand up'. Rising from kneeling to standing (Fig. 6.171) holding crutches or other walking aids to standing and any other rising problems have to be trained in individual children (see Sitting development, rising, p. 133). Fig. 6.172 gives various sequences for rising reactions.

12–18 MONTHS NORMAL DEVELOPMENTAL LEVEL

Common problems

Delay in walking alone, improvement in walking pattern e.g. narrower base, arms coming down from being hold up in abduction, steps more rhythmical, equal, smoother, standing alone and play in standing, rising to standing completely on his own, starting and stopping his walking, stair ascent and descent, use of inclines and walk on rough ground improves until second and third years.

Abnormal performance   A variety of abnormal gait patterns in the walking child, see 'Abnormal Gait' above.

Reflex reactions   The following are expected at this level:
1   Saving from falling by staggering (protective) reactions in lower limbs, forward, sideways, backward, crossing over and hopping; also upper limbs as before.
2   In standing, tilt child backward resulting in trunk flex forward and

dorsiflexion of feet—forward results in back extension, rise onto toes, —laterally results in trunk incurring, inversion of one foot, pronation of the other.

3 Rotate child in standing, feet apart, results in one foot inversion to the rotated side, the other foot in pronation.

Treatment suggestions

Gait   See Figs. 6.160 to 6.164, without support.

Other techniques   See above 9–12 months level but without walking aids.

Stair climbing is also dependent on standing on one leg long enough for the other to deal with the step. This should be trained on and off a low box, progressed to higher boxes as well as staircases, pavements, and ladders.

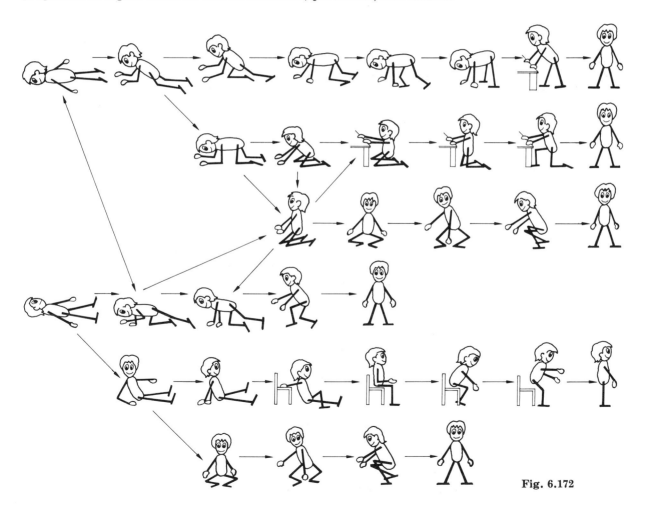

Fig. 6.172

Train walking and stop, walk and turn, walk between and round objects, walk on different terrains.

Train staggering reactions   Hold child's arm and push and pull him in all directions to provoke staggering or hopping reactions (Fig. 6.173). One foot may be held instead and the child pushed forward and a protective step provoked. Also hold hips and sharply rotate child to provide a protective step.

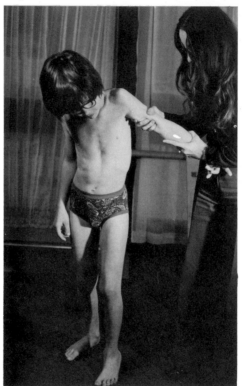

Fig. 6.173

Tilt reactions (Fig. 6.174)   Tilt the child back, side or tilt him at his hips (Fig. 6.175):

—to provoke tilt reaction in trunk with large tilt over.

—to provoke reaction in his feet. See also Chapter 8 on treatment of valgus feet. Carry all these out against manual resistance—'Don't let me push you'.

More advanced counterpoising on one foot is shown using a scooter (Fig. 6.176).

2–7 YEAR LEVELS

Train hop, skip and jump and the variety of activities at the different developmental levels described in the work of Gesell and others (see Table 6.1).

Table 6.1 Motor developmental stages. 2–7 years (based on Gesell, Sheridan, Cratty)

2 years
Climbs onto furniture
Pulls wheeled toy by string
Ascends and descends stairs holding on, two feet per stair
Gait pattern changes from wide base, short, flat foot steps
to narrower base, more heel–toe action established by 3 years
Arms held in abduction during gait come down to relaxed flexion at child's sides
Legs change from external rotation to facing forward
Walk, run AND stops alone
Avoids obstacles while run, or walk, steers wheeled toys
Throws ball without good direction and excessive effort
Arms held out when asked to catch a ball
Walk backwards, sideways, between obstacles
Walks into a ball to attempt kick

2½ years
Jump two feet together
Ascends stairs, holding on, alternate feet
Descends holding on, two feet per stair, ascends two feet no hold
Steers tricycle while 'walking' his feet on ground
Stand and kick ball with one foot
Stand on tip-toe by imitation

3 years
Ascend stairs, no holding on alternate feet
Descend stairs usually two feet per stair, no holding on
Jumps from bottom stair or pavement
Climbing furniture, apparatus well
Run and turn, run and push large toys
Walks on tiptoes, on heels, heel–toe action in walk up inclines, uneven ground
Balance on one foot alone, momentarily, enough to walk on line unsteadily
Pedals tricycles and pedal cars
Imitates movements, e.g. wiggle thumb, asymmetrical arm position unless very complicated

4 years
Throws and catches ball with more control, less effort, more direction and does not need to place arms out to catch
Bounces ball, picks up ball or object with bend from waist
Walk on wide balance beam, near ground, walks heel to toe on line steadily
Stand one one foot 3–5 seconds alone
Hops on right or left foot increasing distance
Imitates finger plays including fine pincer actions
Gait pattern now with arm swing, as adult: stops suddenly. Turn on the spot

5 years
Climbs trees, ladders, apparatus
Expert at sliding, swings 'stunts'
Dances, hop and skip to rhythms
Ball throw and catch in various directions, smaller balls
Kick ball on the run
Counts fingers by pointing

6 years
Wrestle, tumble
Roller skates
Jumps rope, begins skip with rope
Stands on one foot with eyes closed
Bounce and catch balls

Table 6.1   (*contd.*)

7 years
Walks on narrow and high balance bars
Throws ball about 30 feet
Begins team sports

Movement development shows improvement in speed, precision and decrease of effort or extraneous movements. Increase of endurance. Perception of space, timing and rhythm become integrated with many of the motor skills, see Physical education literature for further details and for patterns of performance.

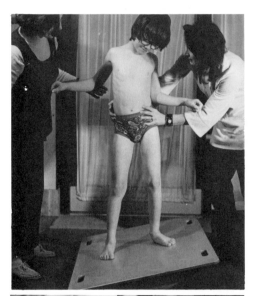

Fig. 6.174

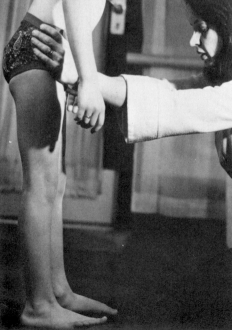

Fig. 6.175

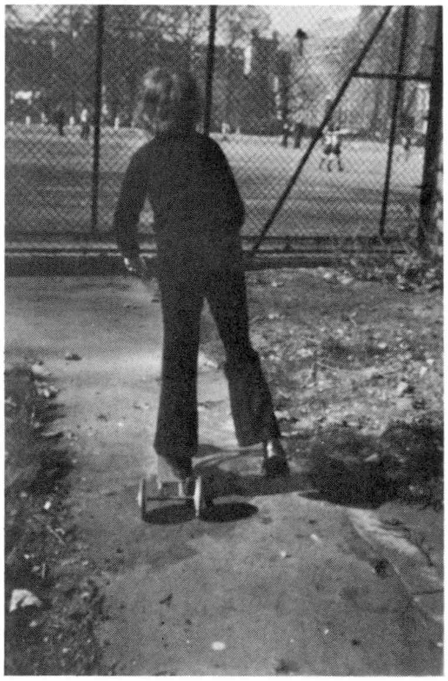

Fig. 6.176

DEVELOPMENT OF HAND FUNCTION

The development of hand function not only depends on the motor control of the shoulder girdle, arms and hands but also on visual, perceptual, perceptual-motor and cognitive development.

The *main motor aspects* of hand function involve the type of grasp, the pattern of reach, the pattern of reach-and-grasp and the pattern of release. These aspects may develop independently of the gross motor activities in prone, supine, sitting, standing and walking development. Although this discrepancy of motor levels appears, it is essential to develop this fine motor ability as:

1 Use of hands is helpful for perceptual development, cognitive development and for the emotional satisfaction of the child.

2 Use of hands is particularly important for the handicapped child for support on open hands or grasp so that he can hold on and sit, stand, walk or pull himself into any position.

3 Hands can be used to help establish shoulder girdle fixation which is fundamental to many of the fine and gross motor skills.

It is, however, impossible to concentrate on hand function without considering the many direct relationships of gross motor development to the acquisition of hand function. These important relationships are:

Upper limbs and the postural mechanisms

1 Establishment of head control is important for hand/eye coordination.

2 Establishment of postural fixation of the shoulder girdle is obtained when leaning on elbows or on hands in various gross motor activities in prone, supine, sitting, standing and walking development. This helps shoulder fixation for reach, reach-and-grasp, and to coordinate manipulation or activities such as pouring liquids.

3 Establishment of head, trunk and pelvic postural fixation and counterpoising in sitting and standing makes it possible to use the hands other than in lying or only if the child is firmly tied to a chair. Thus training of all the counterpoising activities in prone, supine, sitting and standing includes training of reach, reach-and-grasp and release (Fig. 6.177).

4 Development of rising reactions. Hands and arms are used to help in the change of various postures or the assumption of posture in gross motor development.

5 Development of saving reactions in the arms. The upper limbs are thrown into various patterns involving active contractions of the muscles in synergies (patterns), to save and prop the child as he falls off balance.

Although the hands and arms participate in *automatic* saving and propping reactions as well as in various rising reactions, these will not necessarily contribute to *voluntary* movements. Voluntary movements of reach, grasp and release have to be specially trained in fine motor activities.

6 Many of the arm synergies trained in gross motor skills are those used in voluntary reach (Fig. 6.178).

Fig. 6.177 a, Absence of counterpoising in the trunk leads to child falling over the arm during its movement. *Note* Attempts to counterpoise with the better arm or by grasp may occur. Encourage this only if trunk counterpoising is totally impossible. b, The trunk is counterpoising the arm movement. Patterns of arm movements should be trained together with counterpoising, in all positions. *Note* The height of the chair controls the position of the legs. A lower chair should be used to prevent any extensor spasticity, to stabilise the child or diminish athetosis.

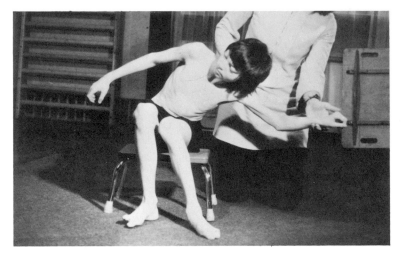

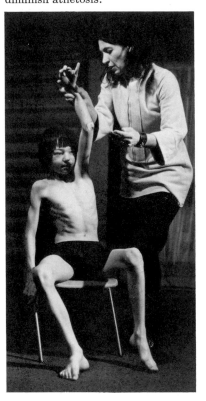

Upper limbs and abnormal motor behaviour

1 Abnormal postures of the whole child include abnormal postures of the arms and hands (Figs. 6.179–6.181). Correction of the whole child, often corrects the arms. Also corrective arm patterns improves the rest of the child (Fig. 6.182).

2 Abnormal reflex reactions in the whole child may prevent or disrupt hand function as well as interfere with achievement of the gross motor abilities.

3 Involuntary movements in the hands or whole arm disrupt hand function. These involuntary movements may stem from the whole body. There may be involuntary motion in another part, say the 'kicking about' of legs only, which disturbs the use of the hands.

Points **1**, **2** and **3**, may all appear in the same child.

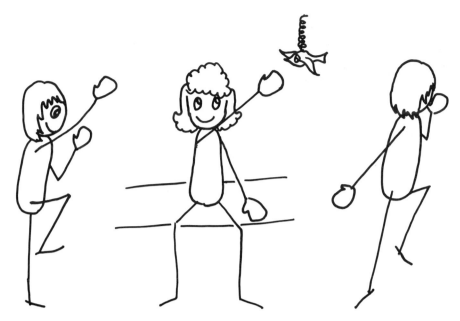

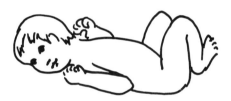

Fig. 6.178 a, Arm pattern of shoulder flexion-adduction-external rotation trained within training of rolling. b, Arm pattern of shoulder flexion-adduction-external rotation as a reaching pattern. c, Arm pattern of shoulder extension-adduction-internal rotation within rolling prone to supine, or within creeping pattern in prone, may be used in reaching back and behind child as, say, in putting on a coat.

Fig. 6.179 Shoulders protracted or retracted with arms flexed-adducted and hands clenched in a predominantly flexed child similar to the newborn. Inability to reach out or can only reach near his body. There is associated difficulty of release if hands flexed on object (grasp).

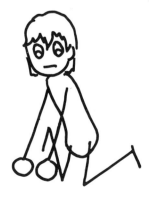

Fig. 6.180 Arms flexed-adducted and internally rotated with elbows flexed and pronated, wrists flexed or mid-position and hands clenched or open. Shoulder flexion-adduction-internal rotation may also occur with elbow extension-pronation. Shoulder flexion-adduction may also occur with elbow supination and flexion in athetoids who 'fold their arms in' towards their bodies in supination, with hands open or clenched.

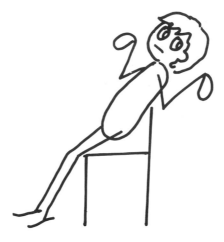

Fig. 6.181 Arms held up in the air in abduction-external rotation, elbow flexion and supination with palms facing toward the child. Elbows may also be flexed and pronated with palms facing outward. Hand may be 'hanging down' or clenched; this is also called the 'bird-wing position' and is seen in supine, sitting and standing positions. There is inability to reach forward, bring hands together and develop 'hand regard' and bring hands down for support.

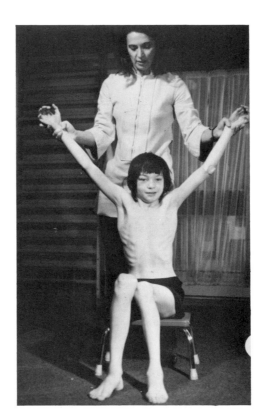

Fig. 6.182 Correction of asymmetry of arms, flexion-adduction-internal rotation and other abnormal postures of the arms also corrects abnormal postures of head and trunk (kyphosis, kyphoscoliosis) and vice versa. *Note* Child must maintain postural fixation in vertical alignment and not fall backward against the therapist.

BASIC ARM AND HAND PATTERNS FOR ALL LEVELS OF DEVELOPMENT

Although one should not be dogmatic about the pattern in which a child uses his arms and hands to achieve his goal, it is important to select corrective patterns below in treatment because (a) abnormal patterns are easier for cerebral palsied children and tend to create deformities which often make movement ineffective and cosmetically unattractive; (b) the child may have no idea on how to move and needs training in basic neuro-muscular patterns. He may later modify these patterns within his individual development.

Abnormal arm patterns and treatment suggestions

Although various arm patterns, or individual joint motions, can be found for correction of abnormal arm patterns, select those which can also be directly related to the use of the arms *in function*. Basic arm patterns which do this are:

1   Shoulder flexion, elbow extension, pronation, hands open or grasp (Fig. 6.183).
2   Diagonal, shoulder elevation-abduction-external rotation, elbow extension or flexion, supination, hands and thumbs open (Fig. 6.184).
3   The opposite diagonal to (2) is down into adduction internal rotation, elbow pronation, hand closed (Fig. 6.185) or open.
4   Diagonal flexion-adduction-external rotation, elbow supination, flexed or extended (Figs. 6.186 and 6.187).
5   The opposite diagonal to (4) is arm extension-abduction-internal rotation (Fig. 6.178), elbow pronation, hand closed, or open (Figs. 6.188 and 6.189).

There are *many variations on the basic patterns* described above.

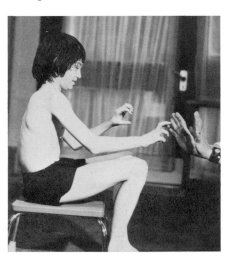

Fig. 6.183 Spastic boy attempting basic pattern of bilateral shoulder flexion with elbow extension and dorsiflexion of the hands. This pattern not only corrects many abnormal patterns as in Figs. 6.179–6.181 but is functionally useful, e.g. shoulder flexion-elbow extension hands flat or grasping support for sitting and standing well; in movements to reach for shoes or socks down at his feet, in pulling off a jumper over his head, reaching down to pull up pants or to push them down to his ankles.

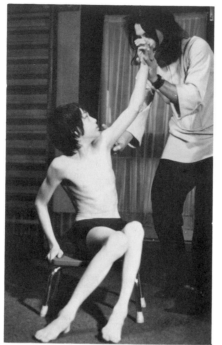

Fig. 6.184

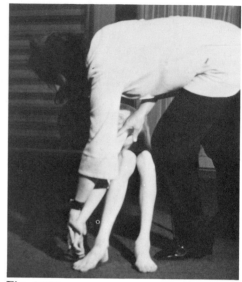

Fig. 6.185

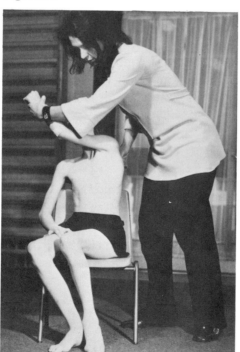

Fig. 6.186

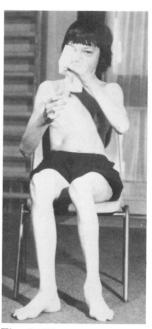

Fig. 6.187

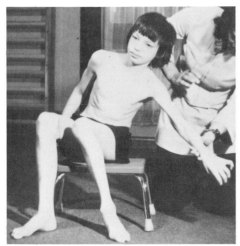

Fig. 6.188

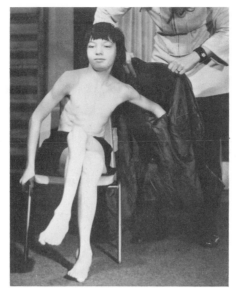

Fig. 6.189

Practical points

Positions Carry out the above patterns in all positions of the child's gross motor levels, i.e. at normal developmental levels of:

0–5 months —use arms in reaching in side-lying, supine, prone on elbows.

5–7 months —arm reach in prone, supine, rolling and then reaching, or arm reaching to roll, sitting propped on hands and reach with one arm.

7–9 months —arm reach on hands and knees, upright kneeling support one forearm on table.

9–12 months—arm reach while sitting independently, upright kneeling or standing *holding* on with one hand.

Over 12 months —arm reach in standing.

Reach and grasp are also carried out in these positions. Trunk rotation with reaching must be included, especially if resistance is given to the child's arm movement.

Direction of reach is first low down in front of child, forward at shoulder level, to the side, above him, and then behind him. This progression is easiest for most children.

Facilitation These patterns can be facilitated with:
1 Touch, pressure stretch and resistance and good rotation of the child's shoulder girdle and/or trunk.
2 The therapist may manually rotate the shoulder girdle, pull shoulders

forward or backward to initiate automatic arm pattern, see Rolling technique (p. 99), Creeping technique (pp. 75, 78).

3 The child can be taught to reach for toys or take part in a play activity selected to provoke the use of specific arm patterns (Fig. 6.183).

4 The child can be asked to concentrate on the arm patterns. e.g. 'stretch your arm up and back', 'stretch your elbow'.

5 The daily activities of feeding, dressing, washing, bathing may use many desirable arm patterns including those described below, if activities are carefully trained.

Vision and arm patterns It is important to stimulate the child's visual development and to associate it with development of hand functions, e.g. encourage child to look at hands or object he is reaching for during facilitation of arm patterns.

Unilateral and bilateral arm patterns must be included in the programme. For example:

1 Unilateral patterns such as moving one side only; leaning on one hand and move with the other; grasp a support with one hand and move the other (assymetrical work) (Figs. 6.184–6.189).

2 Bilateral patterns with the child's arms in the same direction (bilateral and symmetrical) for support and for motion. This takes place to counteract abnormal asymmetry of posture of arms and body, and of function (Figs. 6.190, 6.191 and 6.192, see also Fig. 6.182). Use of less affected arm together with affected arm may help the latter.

3 Bilateral patterns with arm, in opposite directions (bilateral and reciprocal). This takes place in creeping, reciprocal arm swing, or motion using play equipment, pulleys or hand pedals.

4 Bilateral patterns with each arm in a different direction, e.g. one sideways the other forward (bilateral and asymmetrical) which is used in advanced perceptual-motor training and for highly complicated counterpoising activities and hand skills.

Fig. 6.190 Both arms stretch towards toys and palms face inwards to hold toys. In this way elbow extension, supination is correcting the abnormal postures.
Note The rest of the body is also correcting abnormal postures associated with abnormal arm postures.

Use of *both* arms corrects asymmetrical ability in arm function as in hemiplegia.

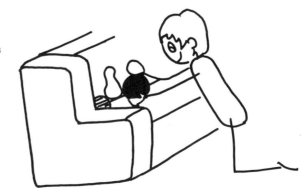

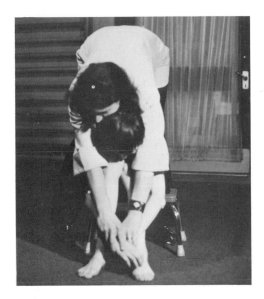

Fig. 6.191

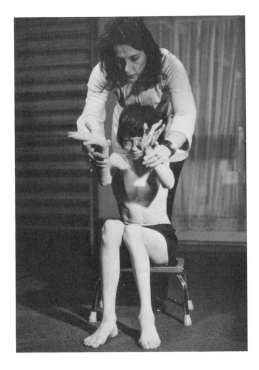

Fig. 6.192

Abnormal hand grasps and treatment suggestions

1 Abnormal grasp may be present in association with the total abnormal posture or only with the arm posture when the rest of the body functions well.

2 Grasp may appear to be abnormal because it belongs to a lower level of development.

Treatment suggestions for some abnormal grasps

Grasp only possible in one position of the child's arm   Train grasp within all the corrective arm patterns (above, in different directions, and body positions).

Wrist flexion with palmer or pincer grasp or inability to grasp in this position (Fig. 6.193) Press the child's wrist down as he tries to grasp;

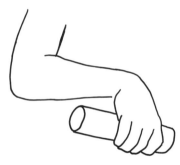

Fig. 6.193

place the object above the level of his wrist; ask him to lift his hands to the object, see Figs. 6.192 and 6.195. Some children may need a wrist splint to train grasp with wrist in extension (dorsiflexion). However, in some spastic children, the wrist extension should only be to the midposition as there is excessively tight finger flexion with full wrist extension. This also prevents the child from opening his hands to release the object held. The use of glove puppets, hammering, lifting dowels out of holes, rings off a stick and similar activities may help to obtain wrist extension for grasp and release. In some cases, grasping with the wrist in extension may be achieved at the cost of opening the hand in this particular position. The child may then discover he can open his hand if he palmer flexes. It is preferable to train hand opening correctly, see below, 0–3 months level, and later release, 9–12 months level.

Excessive finger flexion in grasp   With or without hyperextension of the metacarpophalangeal m-p joints (Fig. 6.194). Place the child's hand over thick, larger objects such as bars and handles. Do not use squeezy toys. Hold the dorsum of the child's hand, lift his m-p joints and he or you can then press his fingers straight over the large ball, box or square bar.

This may be done with the child's m-p joints pressing on the edge of a table as he tries to hold onto the edge, or the solid edge of a truck or windowsill. Counteracting this abnormal grasp will prepare him for grasp with his fingers straight, using finger tips later. Grasping edges of cards or lids is one way of training this straight finger grasp.

Adducted thumbs and ulnar grasp The adducted thumb may grasp or be useless. It can be seen with ulnar grasp (Fig. 6.193). In some children the ulnar grasp may result when the child tries to compensate for or avoid the adducted thumb. When the thumb is abducted a radial grasp may occur.

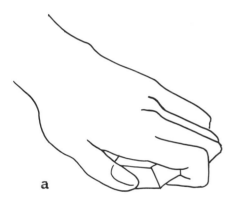
a

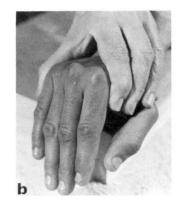
b

Fig. 6.194

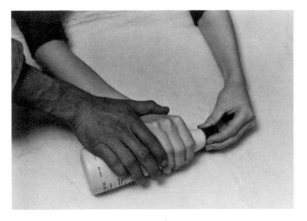

Fig. 6.195

In other cases, the child grasps his fingers in midposition with an adducted thumb. Adducted thumbs may also accompany palmar flexion, or excessive finger flexion with hyperextended m-p joints. The child should be encouraged to move his hand towards the thumb side e.g. he pushes rolling toys away towards the radial side; brings a spoonful of food towards his mouth and other activities which encourage him to move his hand towards the thumb

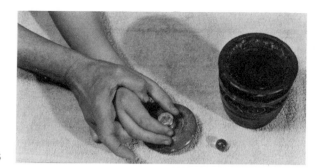

Fig. 6.196

side. He may not manage this unless you hold his hand in midline during grasp. Hold the child's hand between his thumb and forefinger on one side and hold down the ulnar side as he grasps (Fig. 6.196).

The little finger and ring finger may be bandaged if the child does not resent such a procedure. Training grasping of objects with the radial side is then encouraged. Check that the child is not given handgrips on walkers, handles and other supports which encourage an abnormal ulnar grasp. The handles at the sides of rollators or on crutches may do this. Avoid the angled spoons for handicapped children as they create an ulnar grasp. The child's adducted thumb may be abducted-extended if he tries the above suggestions. Also use Techniques for hand opening, Figs. 6.182–6.184, 6.188 and 6.192.

Adducted thumbs may be held out with thumb-splints made from pigskin or other splints (see Appendix). To get an adducted thumb out of a fist or hand, never pull it by its tip or you may dislocate or sublux the m-p joint. Sometimes the other fingers flex more as you do pull on the thumb. Rather turn the whole arm or forearm to face palm up to the ceiling and abduct the thumb out from its base. It is important to follow this procedure with placing the child's hand over a toy teaching him a palmar grasp or later a radial grasp. See Hand opening techniques, p. 188.

Inability to grasp with both hands simultaneously Although this is normal in many children under the 6 months developmental level, it may also be due to:

1 Lack of head control in midline so the child uses the hand that he can see; lack of midline head control is seen in persistent head turning to one side, which occasionally improves spontaneously.

2 Asymmetrical tonic neck response to one side which is 'used' to reach and grasp to that side.

3 Hemiplegia or greater spasticity or weakness of one arm in any diagnostic type.

4 Excessive spasms or involuntary motion on one side, rare hemiathetoids.

5 Sensory loss on one side especially astereognosis in the hand or visual field defect, usually in some hemiplegias.

Inability to grasp on one side will often be associated with *inability to use both hands together* or to hold with one hand and carry out an action with the other. During training of prone, supine, sitting and standing development check that both hands are given objects to grasp simultaneously or to grip for support. Use play activities which require two hands, e.g. play in water and washing, sand, clay, dough, larger toys, handles on bowls, rolling pins, sieves, sticks with dangling bells, broom, bicycle pump, toy concertina, small cymbals, morracas or toys which make a noise if pushed at both ends (Fig. 6.197).

Associated grasping or clenching on the affected side when grasping with the unaffected or the less affected side. This is usually seen in spastic children; associated 'mirror' movements of the hand not in use are normally seen in very young children but disappear on normal development. If these mechanisms persist they can prevent the child's transfer of objects from hand to hand and holding with one hand while using the other hand. Hold the more affected elbow straight with hand flat on the table while the other hand grasps. Have the child lean on the more affected hand held open, with the weight on the elbow or hand. Carry out joint compression to facilitate support on this hand as the other hand is used actively. Practise activities which include each hand in a different action, e.g. hold toy with one hand, carry out action with the other, winding a bandage or hold support with one hand and use a variety of movements with the other.

Other parts of the body may also tense or assume abnormal postures during grasp. Check that these associated reactions are corrected as well. Correct positioning of the rest of the body during hand function will control this.

Practical points in training grasp

1 Use of the eyes must be associated with development of hand function. Follow the developmental levels below.

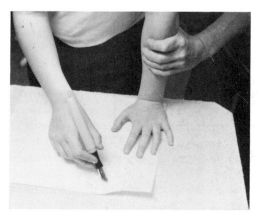

Fig. 6.197

2 Normally the grasp reflex and hand clenching disappear before voluntary grasp develops. Do not wait or work on total disappearance before putting the object in the child's hand to grasp. Use techniques (below) to open the hand just before methods to develop palmar grasp, in the same session.

3 Children should not grasp in association with any of the abnormal arm postures shown in Figs. 6.179–6.181 e.g. grasp with wrist and/or elbow flexed, shoulder adducted and flexed. Use the arm patterns suggested in **Basic arm and hand patterns**, p. 173. Check that the rest of his body does not assume abnormal postures as he grasps.

4 Have the child hold objects with his hand in pronation, then later in midposition and still later in supination. However, some athetoid children may start with grasp in supination and then midposition and finally in pronation.

5 Make sure that the child looks at the object in his hand. Talk about the object at his comprehension level. Encourage his speech during the use of his hands.

6 Check that he is interested in the choice of object placed in his hand.

Abnormal release and treatment suggestions

Total inability to let go of an object placed or grasped by the child after 5 months.

Release only possible if wrist is flexed   The child may use his other hand, his chin or even his forehead, or a hard surface to press the back of his hand to obtain this flexion (palmar flexion).

Release against a hard surface after 11 months of age. These problems of release are discussed in the appropriate developmental levels below.

Release with thumb adducted and flexed in palm   Train a release with thumb abduction with a supinated forearm. Sometimes external rotation from the shoulder is indicated. Thumb splints may help. Movements to train hand opening also contribute to keeping the thumb out of the palm. Supination of the child's forearm by the therapist facilitates thumb extension or abduction.

Release with ulnar deviation can be improved if objects are released into container or dowel holes on the radial side of the hand.

Release with excessive splaying of the fingers, i.e. hyperabduction with hyperextended metacarpalphalangeal joint. A similar pattern is also seen in normal babies casting objects at about 11–15 months of age. In addition this pattern is seen in avoiding reactions in the hands of athetoid children. There may also be plantar and/or a visual avoiding reaction with the avoiding reaction in the hands caused by tactile and visual stimuli respectively. Grasp smaller objects and train release into a defined area or container. Hold the ulnar side of the child's hand and train release on the radial side and later with thumb and finger. Training more precise release is closely allied with the training of pincer grasp below (Fig. 6.196).

Hand and visual avoiding reactions can be helped if one introduces the object for grasp and release slowly into the child's visual field and into his hands. Encourage him to maintain his grasp to make him less sensitive to the stimuli.

Conflict between grasp and release This problem is seen in an athetoid child when he makes attempts to grasp an object but immediately withdraws his hand, splaying it open as in the pattern in (6) above. This presents itself as a repeated involuntary motion in the hands. This conflict between the grasp reflex and the avoiding reactions was described by Denny-Browne and Twitchell [92]. To break this disabling conflict, it is advisable to reinforce the child's active grasp or grip. Encourage maintained grasp for as much of the day as possible on bars, handles, in front, at his side, above or below him in his various situations during the day. When he is sitting on a pot he should grasp a bar, sitting in a pram, he should grasp a bar, standing and using walkers or hold sticks vertically or frequently carry around a rod grasped in both or one hand.

Other involuntary motion disrupting reach and grasp Train conscious control of reach, grasp and manipulation. With practice the involuntary motion decreases. Help the child by having him use his hands while leaning on his forearms, or reach to toys through a thin padded hoop which limits the excursion of the involuntary motion. Wide uprights of, say, a play pen also limit his involuntary motion as he reaches between them for toys.

Note It is important to carry out all the training of reach, grasp and release as suggested below under the appropriate developmental levels. The patterns of reach, grasp and release may only be retarded in some children. This means the pattern may be a normal one but seen at an earlier age than the child's chronological age as in mentally subnormal children.

All the patterns of grasp and release are also disrupted by visual loss, any sensory loss in the hands, as say in hemiplegia, and by lack of visual, perceptual or perceptual-motor development as in intelligent 'clumsy' children.

STAGES OF HAND FUNCTION DEVELOPMENT

0–3 MONTHS NORMAL DEVELOPMENTAL LEVEL

Common problems

Delay in eye focussing, visual fixation, visual following of an object. Clenched hands not opening; thumb still held in palm.

Abnormal performance, see abnormal patterns of arms and hand above.

Reflex reactions Grasp reflex, Moro reaction, tonic neck reaction, sudden flexor or extensor spasms.

Treatment suggestions and daily care

Eye focus and following (hearing-and-vision)
1   First offer visual interest in the midline and help the child keep his head in midline. You may need to hold both his shoulders forward, occasionally backward to allow him to keep his head upright (see Sitting Development, vertical head control, Prone Development, head control).
2   At first place your face, or toys close to the child's eyes, about 8″ from him.
3   Eye-to-eye contact is of first importance before interest in objects. This should be done at the child's eye level whether he is in side-lying, supine, prone, supported sitting or supported standing.
4   Associate vision, hearing and head control with face-to-face singing, talking. Vary tones of voice. Encourage baby's smile and general communication.
5   Help him to look at and follow shiny, moving, colourful noise making mobiles, toys, fishes in a tank, marble runs, a torch light, switching the room light on and off. Use coloured ribbons, Christmas decorations, shiny milk tops or other bottle tops strung together, rattles.
6   Use red, yellow or primary colours, not pastels.
7   Use jingling noises and not high pitched or sudden loud noises as the child may still have a startle reflex.
8   Hang tinkling bells or jingling beads or mobiles in the window or doorway so that they move and make a sound as the wind blows or if they are touched by you or by his early crude arm reaching movements at 5 months level.
9   Encourage the child to look and see where the noise came from, to listen to your voice. Put him in different positions, i.e. prop the child up in sitting as well as lying on his back, side or stomach to carry out the above.

DEVELOPMENT OF HAND FUNCTION AND EYE–HAND COORDINATION (Table 6.2)

Table 6.2 Development of hand function and eye–hand coordination

0–3 months
  Eye-to-eye contact (parallel eyes).
  Fix eyes on light; eyes follow object to midline (1 month), to past midline (2 months) over 180 degrees (3 months), down, then up eye movement.
  Hands opening from closed posture.
  REFLEX REACTIONS: Tactile grasp; stretch grasp; blink; doll's eye reflex. Moro, ATNR.

3–5 months
  'Grasp with his eyes' when interested in object.
  'Hand regard' or studies his hands, bring hands together in midline, clutch and unclutches hands.
  Visual exploration of environment.
  Clumsy reaching attempts.
  Clutches clothes, touches body, mouth, face.
  Grasps object placed in hand.
  REFLEX REACTIONS: Moro, ATNR disappearing, absence of grasp reflex.

5–7 months
  Reaching successfully in all directions, depending on trunk balance.
  Bilateral reach becomes unilateral reach by 7 months.
  Grasp feet in supine and sitting–bilateral then unilateral.
  Maintained grasp (grip)—while sitting.
  Ulnar grasp changing to palmar grasp.
  Mirror movements of grasp in the other hand.
  Moves head to see things, eyes converge and focus on pellet at 10 feet. Smaller pellets seen by 9 months (Stycar tests).
  Continues to mouth everything, hand to mouth movement.
  REFLEX REACTIONS: Saving and propping downward, forward and beginning laterally.

7–9 months
  Transfer object from hand to hand.
  Unilateral reach and grasp.
  Radial grasp, beginning use of fingertips.
  Holds one block while given another.
  Offers cube, but cannot release it.
  Releases cube by pressing it against a hard surface.
  Bangs two objects together.
  Pats, bangs, strokes, clutches, rakes, scratches—pats mother's face, pats image of face in mirror.

9–12 months
  Protrudes index finger, pokes objects with finger.
  Grasps between fingers and thumb then one finger and thumb (crude to fine pincer grasp).
  Achieving dynamic tripod between thumb index and middle finger for scribbling with pencil.
  Reach and grasp possible in all directions, with supination and other improved control of arm.

Release with gross opening of hand then more precise until places small objects in jar, peg in hole, etc.
Looks for fallen toy.

12–15 months
Casting of toys stopping.
Watches small toy moved across room up to 12 feet.
Builds tower of two cubes.
Pushes and pulls large toys.
Drinks alone from cup, often spills.

18 months to one year
Delicate pincer grasp.
Takes off shoes, socks.
Turns pages of book.
Strings large beads later smaller beads.
Scribbles with pencil.
Feeds self clumsily.
Hand preference more obvious.

2 years
Increasing finer movements.
Throws ball accurately.
Unwraps sweet.
Screws and unscrews lids, toys.
Imitate vertical line; scribbles and dots.

3 years
Takes off all clothes
Feeds self completely, using fork.
Copies circle.
Draws a man simply.
Cuts with scissors.
Washes alone.

4 years
Draws simple house, more detailed man.
Brushes teeth, dresses alone except for buttons and laces.
Constructive building include three steps with cubes.
Matches and names four colours.
Copies cross.

5 years
Copies square, triangle, letters.
Matches 12 colours.
Drawing and copying improved.
Use knife and fork.
Dresses and undresses completely.

Note Many conceptual and perceptual abilities are omitted, and are usually found under mental development, but are also interwoven with hand function (see also: Development of Feeding, Dressing, Perception in Chapter 7).

Also see 'Opening of hand', treatment suggestions below and in other motor developmental training, for example:

1   Hand may open within the arm pattern of elevation-abduction-external rotation, or extension-adduction-internal rotation in techniques of creeping, or used later in prone development, in supine, side-lying, sitting or standing (Figs. 6.178, 6.182–184, 6.188 and 6.192).

2   Weight bearing on elbows and/or on hands decreases hand clenching, see prone, sitting, standing development which include leaning on elbows or hands.

3   See Correction of postures in all developmental levels—as these also correct arms and hands.

3–5 MONTHS NORMAL DEVELOPMENTAL LEVEL

Common problems

Delay in 'hand regard', visual exploration; bring hands together and to mouth, touching self, unable to grasp object placed in hand, grasp and shake toy, no clumsy reaching for objects. Grasp is normally on ulnar side at this level. Clutches clothes of self or mother may be delayed.

Abnormal performance

1   Asymmetrical bringing of hands to midline, reach or grasp.

2   Touching with semiflexed or closed hand.

3   Abnormal patterns in reaching (see abnormal patterns, arms and hands above).

4   Abnormal grasp (see above) except ulnar or lateral grasp.

Treatment suggestions and daily care

Hand regard and bringing hands to midline   Positions to bring arms forward are:

1   Place the child in side-lying or lying in a hammock, or half-lying in a sack of polystyrene beads, with shoulders brought forward or in supported sitting with arms held forward or if possible sitting and leaning with his body against the table or your lap, his arms placed well forward. These positions offer more opportunity than supine for bringing his arms to midline level with his eyes. Only in those cases when the child *can* bring his arms forward is it advisable to have him in supine. A side-lying board is helpful for those children who persist in keeping their arms in abnormal positions at their sides, out of their view (see Supine Development, p. 106).

2   Once his hands are in front of him the child should be made aware of them by your talk, shining a torch on them, putting sticky things such as

jam on his hands, playing with his fingers, putting thimbles, rings, coloured ribbon, bracelets or bells on his wrist and fingers. Help him open his hands and rub his palms together, touch his face and body and later clasp and unclasp hands, clutch materials and toys which are soft and easy to clutch.

Opening of hand
1   Stimulate the child's whole palm by rubbing it with rough textures, especially sand, during play activities.
2   Rhythmical shake of the child's arm from his shoulder.
3   Stroke the ulnar surface of his hand and little finger.
4   You or the child press the 'heel' of his hand on a firm surface especially combined with your giving pressure (joint compression) through a straight shoulder and extended elbow (p. 82, Prone development).
5   Holding the child's upper arms and turning them outwards, in some cases you only need to turn the elbow, so that the palm faces up. The child should do this himself as far as he can to hold a toy, ball or see a picture drawn on his hand. See other arm patterns in Figs. above.
6   Have the child's arms well away from his body. This avoids hand clenching in some children. Open the child's hand over a large rubber, wooden or plastic object. DO NOT give toys which stimulate clenching, such as squeezy toys. Do not have objects too big for his small hands. Grasping a cone with the large end on the side of his little finger helps to overcome hand clenching.
7   Open hands when child is prone leaning on elbows or hands, on hands and knees, sitting lean on hands, standing lean on hands. Open his hands by any of the above methods pressing the 'heel' of the hand down. Pull the thumb or fingers out from the base and not from their tips.

Hand grasp
1   See above suggestions for treating abnormal grasp.
2   Place large objects in the child's hands, e.g. balls, cylinders, cones, large blocks of a size that fit into the whole palm of his hand. They should not be so small that abnormal clenching occurs. Some children first learn to grasp soft objects more easily than hard ones or vice versa, so try a variety to begin with to find which each child prefers, and then gradually introduce other types.
3   Light objects are often easier than heavy ones.
4   Toys may be teething toys, hoops, tenoquoits, rattles, toy dumb bells, large rings, thick tubing with coloured liquid inside, cotton reels, sponge rubber toys. Avoid squeezy toys if he is very spastic.
5   Place his hands around large hand grips, handles, bars so that as a result he can sit up, kneel up or stand up or enjoy a ride on a swing, rocking horse or see-saw.
6   Thicken handles of spoons, pencils, toys with rubber hardened clay, wood, a rubber ball or cotton reels, attach hands from, say screw drivers.

7 Encourage the child to hold rusks or spoon in feeding. Hold his hand on the spoon handle. Encourage him to hold a piece of his clothing as you help him undress; to hold his sponge in the bath, or hold his wet wash-cloth.

Besides placing objects of different shapes in his hand make sure to place other objects of different sensation into his hands, e.g. beanbags, fur, velvet and suede objects, sandpaper, crinkling chocolate paper, shoe brushes, wooden, metal and plastic objects. Use sand and water, dough, clay and modelling materials. Name these sensations for him as he feels them.

Help him to grasp and bring objects to his mouth to suck, lick, bite or chew, or to his nose to smell. Develop *grasp-and-squeeze*, sponge in bath, or large woollen pom-pom; *grasp-and-shake* a toy, rattle or morracas, *grasp-and-wave* a toy flag, ribbons, bells. *Grasp-and-drop* is present but it is not grasp and release which develops later (11 months). Grasp-and-push, grasp-and-pull, grasp-and-place and a variety of types of grasps also develop later (Fig. 6.199).

5–7 MONTHS NORMAL DEVELOPMENTAL LEVEL

Common problems

Delay in successful reaching in all or one direction, voluntary grip, palmar grasp, and manipulation of object in his hand, reach-and-grasp, taking weight on hands. Dropping of the object is normal but by 7 months he should hold a second block in the same hand and not drop the first. Delay in hand-to-mouth activities to 'mouth' everything; in bilateral then unilateral grasp of his feet, play with his toes.

Abnormal performance   As in 3–5 months level (see above).

Reflex reactions
1 Saving reaction in arms down and forward is expected.
2 Abnormal persistence of reflex reactions from earlier levels.

Treatment suggestions and daily care

1 See above for reach and for grasp.
2 Continue 0–5 months but combine reach-*and*-grasp.
3 Continue as above expecting the child to do more on his own. Expect him to combine reach and grasp alone. See 6–9 months level in Prone development, for taking weight on hands: used also in sitting and standing development. See also stimulation of saving reactions in Prone Sitting and Standing Development.

7–9 MONTHS NORMAL DEVELOPMENTAL LEVEL

Common problems

Delay in transfer from hand to hand, unilateral reach-and-grasp, grasp more than one block at a time, radial grasp, hand patting, banging, clutch, stroke, rake, scratch, bang two blocks together, release against a hard surface, use of hands in feeding and in holding on during sitting and standing. 'Scissors' grasp (inferior pincer grasp) and use of fingertips.

Reflex reactions
1   Saving and propping reactions expected.
2   Abnormal persistence of reactions from previous levels.

Treatment suggestions and daily care

1   See above for reach and grasp patterns.
2   Train own grasp in feeding, dressing, washing, toileting (Chapter 7). Begin training release by having the child release a block against a hard surface with the heel of his hand held down against the surface, or his other hand or his body. Release may be impossible if hand opening has not yet been developed. See methods at 0–5 months level or training of hand opening.
3   Ulnar grasp should develop into radial grasp.
4   Transfer from hand to hand, banging blocks together and holding on with one hand or leaning on one hand during unilateral reaching are particularly important for hemiplegic children, and any child with asymmetrical postures.
5   Play with suitable toys, dough, sand, water can involve transfer from hand to hand, grasp more than one object at a time as well as patting, banging, clutching, stroking, raking, scratching and release against a hard surface.
6   Patting with open hands may become a persistent pattern in some mentally subnormal children and should be diminished with activities involving grasp and manipulation at the child's developmental level.

9–12 MONTHS NORMAL DEVELOPMENTAL LEVEL

Common problems

Delay in finger/thumb opposition and development of crude and fine pincer grasp, no protrusion of index finger. Release of objects, casting, haphazardly and delay of increasing control into containers, building 2 cube tower, look for fallen toy (permanence of objects). Supination may not develop.

Abnormal performance   See abnormal arm posture, abnormal reach and grasp (above). Abnormal arm patterns prevent increasing control of shoulder, elbow and hand. Abnormal grasp prevents pincer grasp, and index finger approach.

Reflex reactions
1   Excessive avoiding reaction may prevent release becoming controlled as well as preventing grasp (casting toys is normal at this level of development).
2   Saving and propping backwards is expected at this level.

Treatment suggestions and daily care

1   See training of reach and grasp especially grasp in supination.

Index finger approach to objects; isolated finger pointing and pressing.
1   Help the child to use toy telephones or ordinary telephones, using his index finger for dialling.
2   Use index finger to press into dough, plasticine or sand. Later make lines and scribbles in sand.
3   Put paint on finger tip and make dots and scribbles.
4   Press studs on clothes should be attempted. Press small button or knob which obtain interesting sound or visual appearance as say a jack-in-the-box or other pop-up toys. Help him switch electric lights on.
5   Use finger puppets.
6   Play the keys of a piano, typewriter, cash register or with an abacus.

Pincer Grasp   Begin with larger objects then progress to smaller objects. Thumbs and all finger tips are used first before thumb and one finger, usually the index is used. (Crude and fine pincer grasp.)

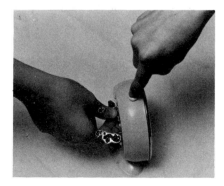

Fig. 6.198

1   Pick up small sweets and place in container or in his mouth. The child should pick up buttons, wooden beads, marbles, under supervision as he may pop them into his mouth to swallow them.

2   Hold thick crayons and if possible pencils and thick chalk for making marks on paper or later writing (Fig. 6.197).

3   Use toys with small knobs and of small size for fitting shapes.

4   Hold small cup handles for drinking.

5   Wind clock and turn its knobs, press alarm bell to stop, press doorbells. Various toys have knobs and buttons to press and turn.

6.   Begin screwing action with large screw-toys, lids, etc (Figs. 6.195, 6.198); progress to medium and fine screwing later.

Allow the child to attempt the activities on his own. If he cannot manage to isolate his index finger, hold his little, ring and middle finger flexed for him until he can do this alone (Fig. 6.196).

Use 'finger plays' for index finger and touch finger to thumb games. 'Make spectacles', blow soap bubbles, 'say how do you do' and 'walk' fingers.

Develop a greater variety of grasps (Fig. 6.199).

Continue training release   This involves dropping of objects (beanbags) in container on the ground below his chair, in front of his chair, at the side and behind his chair. Help him look and see 'where it dropped'. Later encourage him to place small objects in smaller containers until he learns to fit a peg in a formboard, and build one block on top of the other. Precise release is required for building a tower of blocks as well as perceptual and conceptual adequacy. Building blocks may be made of sponge rubber shapes, wood, plastic or be household objects, boxes, tins or pots, to develop the child at this level.

Manipulation and perception/conception   Manipulation is by now integrated with perceptual development of:

Fig 6.199. *Some hand grasps* to take hold of and to grip.
Spherical with palm or fingertips only, Hook grasp, Cylindrical grasp. Others are Lumbrical Fig. 6.195, Pincer Figs. 6.196, 6.197 with sides and with tips of fingers. *Remember* to:
Train grasps in vertical, pronated, supinated and other hand positions.

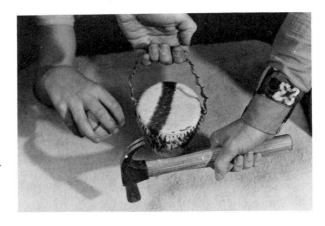

1   Space and depth in, say, well coordinated reach and grasp activities.
2   Form in placing a round peg in a round hole and similar matching.
3   Size in placing small objects into large containers, arrange according to size etc.
4   Colour and shape in use of matching toys (but not naming them), such as various posting boxes, mosaics and other sorting activities, jigsaws.
5   Discrimination of soft, hard, scratchy, smooth sensations.
6   Other conceptions in social activities; wave bye-bye, point to visual stimulus, pat own face in mirror and smile at himself, and plays 'pat-a-cake'.

Perception, conception and fine motor manipulation continues to develop in such activities as threading large beads, smaller beads, other threading toys, scribbling, drawing, painting, pasting, using pegboards, draughts, jigsaws with knobs, sorting buttons, shells, using sewing cards, and a large variety of constructional toys, screwing toys, posting boxes and many more suggested in toy catalogues and by the Toy Libraries Association. Eye-hand co-ordination and rhythm, speed and precision of movement should be developed further after the basic arm and hand actions are trained [106–112] (see Appendix).

CHAPTER 7

MOTOR FUNCTION AND
THE CHILD'S DAILY LIFE

Chapter 6 has presented ways in which the child may develop various postures, maintain these postures during movement, or disturbance of balance, get in and out of postures, obtain various forms of locomotion, and acquire the use of his hands. All these motor functions are used in the child's daily life and a few are summarised to demonstrate their use in self-care, perception, speech and language and socialisation. The child's mental and emotional development is also involved in that they influence the ability to acquire the motor functions which are needed. Alternatively the achievement of motor functions assists this development.

MOTOR FUNCTION AND FEEDING, DRESSING, TOILETTING, WASHING, BATHING, PLAY AND COMMUNICATION

Those below are of particular significance although all motor functions are needed.

Vertical head control in midline and slightly forward.

Obtained by: Holding the child's shoulders forward with your arm when he sits on your lap when a baby; or next to you on his chair when older. Facing the child and holding his arms stretched forward across the table between you or holding him in weight bearing on his forearms. With his grasp and trunk leaning against the table or forearm support the child may do this alone.

This is especially needed for being fed, feeding himself, communication, visual exploration and other functions.

Sitting on the floor and/or sitting on a chair of the correct size and design

Obtained by: Sitting, leaning trunk against table, box or pouffe or other support, leaning on forearms and feeding, drinking, washing his face, playing, pulling off a jumper and so on (Fig. 7.1). Support is also possible by having the child grasp a rail or horizontal bar attached to the table, the wall, the bath, the toy shelves during daily activities (Fig. 7.2). Sitting astride his own chair and grasping its rungs may also be useful for com-

194

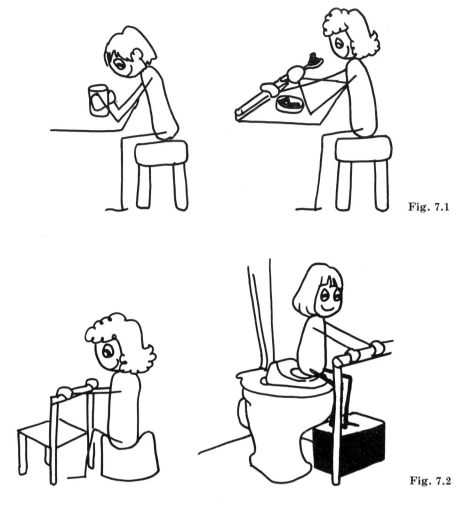

Fig. 7.1

Fig. 7.2

munication, play, dressing and feeding. The child's one arm may be released for any activity, whilst his other controls his balance. Support may be needed for some children from behind by an adult sitting there and holding the child forward with her own body or her hand or by stabilising the child's pelvis with her knees, or with her feet and knees if she is sitting at a higher level to the child.

Sitting with support to the child's pelvis may be carried out with groin straps, diagonal strap across the hips or by firm pressure with your hand in the lower area of the child's back, or holding his hips. The child can then carry out any particular activity using head, trunk and hand control. Sitting against a wall, in a room corner or on a variety of chairs may be used for particular children. Do not let the child slump or slide down during activities.

Correction of abnormal postures are needed so that the child can function (Fig. 7.3).

Prone and head control is used for play, communication, or when being washed, dressed or having a nappy changed in babyhood. Some use this for chewing, sucking and swallowing to increase action of the muscles against gravity.
Obtained by: Use of wedges, rolls, over your arms or lap.

Standing or kneeling upright, holding onto tables, rails for painting, drawing, washing, toilet for boys, dressing, communication and many other play activities.
   Obtained by: Use of horizontal sometimes vertical rails on tables, walls, blackboards, easels, leaning against stable furniture, holding rungs of a chair or use of various standing frames, prone boards attached to tables.

'*On hands and knees*' may be needed for play with cars and trains, gardening, housekeeping activities, sandpits, painting.
   Obtained by: Cushions, wedge cut out to fit a child, over adult's lap when sitting on the floor, or have the child on a crawler which is stabilised.

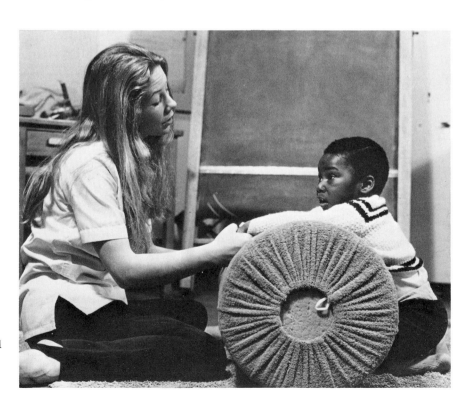

Fig. 7.3 Speech therapy associated with control of excessive extensor thrusts of head, trunk and legs, asymmetry by correct position. Vertical head control and face-to-face communication is promoted. Grasp is developed.

This position is *not* advisable for those children who sit back on their heels during the activity or who have tightly bent hips and knees.

Use of the hands is obviously required for all activities and cannot be condensed unless a particular activity is discussed in detail.

MOTOR FUNCTION AND PERCEPTION [106–112]

All the training for motor function is also training perception. Thus during the motor developmental techniques the therapist should recognise and involve the following main features:

Tactile recognition and discrimination of textures, temperatures. Also feeling different shapes, sizes, weights, to develop stereognosis. Meanings of words are also associated with these experiences of say smooth, hard, scratchy, knobbly, rough, hot and cold. Later matching and discriminating of these sensations develops.

Recognition of the child's own body by tactile recognition during motor training as when touching his mouth, face, grasping his foot or clasping his hands, as well as touching others and sitting close to others.

During motor training, communication and other activities the child can learn his body parts by having his nails painted, putting on rings, bells, bracelets, make-up moustaches, earrings, ribbons, bandages, thimbles or lighting up parts of his body with a torch. When handling the child in movement training rub, stroke, or use ice as well as words to draw attention to parts of his body.

Drawing attention to the child's body parts leads to an awareness of his own spatial relationships or body scheme i.e. Where are his toes?— in front, below and so on. This is also involved with his body planes (Cratty) and which part of his body is moving and in which direction. Although this is experienced through sensation and proprioception, it need not be made conscious during motor training unless this conscious awareness is helpful to train movement itself or to train perception. This verbal visual and proprioceptive linking is considered of importance by psychologists, teachers and physical educators, for the child's future educational activities.

Intersensory development is encouraged by associating the movements trained with hearing and vision. During the training of hand function there is obviously linking between what the child grasps, feels, sees and even tastes and smells. Manipulation of objects with banging, throwing, squeezing, rolling, mouthing, breaking are linking many senses. This leads to another related perceptual experience, which is:

Appreciation of the qualities of objects and of their relations to one another
With gross motor activity and fine motor activity the child should be helped
to recognise round, square, long, cylindrical shapes and discover which
fits into which, which can be placed on top of which object and also which
object is nearer, further away, or behind, in front of or next to the other.
These perceptions and concepts are part of education and occupational
therapy and must be presented to children through various activities.
Motor training overlaps into these areas.

Appreciation of the child's relationship to objects and space   These perceptual experiences also become involved with motor function. As the child
learns to move through space he is also learning to appreciate how far he
is from objects, how to get into and out of things, how to get on top of,
under, around, behind and many other relationships to objects and space.

Thus the child finds out about his body parts, their relations to each
other and also the relations of his body to objects and to space during
gross motor development and fine motor development.

*Development of praxia, motor planning or using the movements appropriate
to a motor task* such as dressing, writing, using a pair of scissors or other
implements. Although this depends on perceptual experiences and on the
training of the neuromuscular system and is helped in its development
during motor developmental training, it could be defective on its own in
brain damaged children.

Specialised perceptual and praxic training (including visuomotor training)
This may still be needed for many specific problems found amongst motor
handicapped children. These problems occur despite general perceptual
experiences included in the motor developmental training. The specialised
therapy and education needed is discussed elsewhere and advice must be
sought from psychologists, teachers in special education and occupational
therapists [106–112].

Although special sessions of perceptual-motor training are needed it
must be remembered that *perception training is also being trained within
the activities of feeding, dressing, washing, bathing, toiletting and especially
playing*, and is part of the programme.

MOTOR FUNCTION AND SPEECH AND LANGUAGE

All the motor developmental training should be associated with words
related to body parts, movements and the purpose of motor functions.
Colours, shapes, sizes and all the other perceptual and conceptual experiences integrated with motor function is also involved in development of
speech and language.

Motor functions have already been summarised above for positions for communication, for feeding, for play, as well as other daily activities. All this promotes speech and language as well. The development of feeding develops the use of the oral musculature needed for speech. In addition, breathing exercises and stimulation of the facial muscles with neuromuscular techniques of touch, pressure, stretch, and resistance may be helpful. Short periods of ice application, or ice lollies reduces spasticity of tongues or mouths and precedes speech. Quick ice stimulation of the mouth muscles may help 'flabby mouths' and make the child aware of his muscles of speech. This discourages dribbling by provoking mouth closure so facilitating swallowing. A large red handkerchief pinned to the child's clothes has motivated some children to remember to wipe their mouths and remember to swallow and keep lips closed. Unobtrusive pressure across the area between nose and upper lip or sometimes just below the lower lip provokes mouth closure and makes swallowing possible, instead of dribbling.

Drooling is normal until about 15 months of age.

The development of speech and language requires special advice and treatment from speech therapists.

Development of communication—brief summary.

(Hearing, speech, language and communication).

0–3 months   Use of cry, facial expression. Stills to noise.

3–4 months   Sounds vary and beginning to babble.

4–6 months   Babbling, begins some intonations. Watches adult's lips. Turns to sounds; to mother's voice. Laughs, squeals, chuckles, annoyed screams.

6–8 months   Lip and tongue sounds. Syllables (baba a ba) begin.

8–12 months   Double syllables, first word. Turns to sounds that interest him instantaneously. Vocalises to make personal contact.

12 months   Understands more than expresses. Follows adult's simple direction ('Give me', 'No'). Responds to his name

12–24 months   Imitates adult speech. Echolalia. 2 or 3 word phrases. Responds and discriminates sounds, speech, simple commands.

3 years   Simple sentences, many questions. Give own name. Nursery rhymes, talks to himself. Normal stutter.

Practical suggestions

1   Follow general guide of developmental levels and individual assessment by speech therapist and psychologist.

2   Always try to communicate with the child with noises (at first not too loud and sudden), songs, smiles, gestures; talk near the child and with face-to-face contact.

3 Speak slowly and distinctly but not with exaggerated articulation, as in 'baby talk'. Wait for any response by the child.

4 Say names of familiar objects, colours, what they are used for, and demonstrate and name parts of the body, and talk of child's own experiences.

5 Child should be able to see your face in a good light during speech. Try to be at his eye level whenever possible.

6 Play lip and tongue games, lick off jam, lollies, peanut butter and during feeding use babbling and speech and stimulate child to do so.

7 Encourage child to participate in songs, rhythms, body movements and hand finger plays. However do not pressurise the child to speak but create informal situations for conversation especially in groups.

8 Use gestures, facial expressions, but not if speech is possible. Make it rewarding for him to use speech or have a need for speech by having to ask for things, indicate things and so on.

9 Praise but do not fuss about the child's attempts to speak and give him time to express himself. Do not finish sentences for him if he can do so in his own time. Do not answer for him if he can say something.

Development of feeding—brief summary

0–4 months Rooting reaction, sucking-and-swallowing reflex. Hypersensitive mouth or cardinal points reflexes, tongue thrust, open mouth and dribbling.

4–6 months Sucking dissociates from swallowing as child transfers liquids for swallowing. All reflexes disappeared. Bite reflex weak. Takes liquids from spoon. Recognises bottle.

6–9 months Takes strained foods, solids, bites a biscuit. Holds a biscuit, may crumble in his hand. Up and down jaw motion in chewing, swallows with mouth closed.

9–12 months Finger feeds, chewing with lateral jaw motion, holds and drinks from bottle, from cup with help. Helps mother with spoon to mouth.

9–12 months Holds spoon alone but cannot bring to mouth with food.

12–15 months Uses spoon but turns it upside down before reaching mouth or within mouth.

Holds and drinks from cup, often spills.

15–18 months Chewing established. Forward and rotary jaw motion. Feeds self clumsily.

2 years Uses spoon correctly, occasional spilling, holds glass and cup for drinking, plays with food. Understand what is edible and inedible. Begins straw drinking but bites edge.

2–3 years Feeds self completely with spoon, with fork. Pours liquids, obtains own drink from tap.

3–4 years Serves self at table, spreads butter, cuts food.

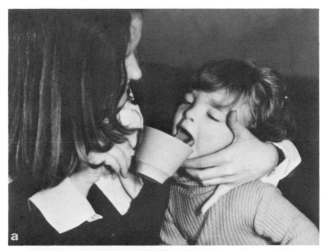

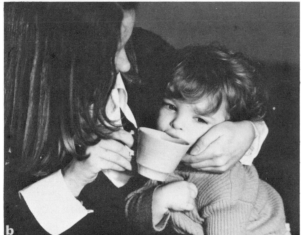

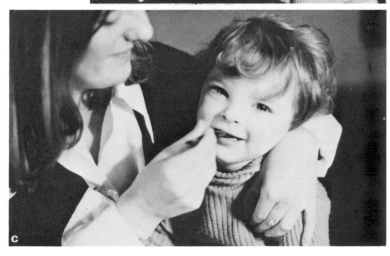

Fig. 7.4 a, Head extension and tongue thrust interfering with drinking and eating. b, Holding the child's head upright and forward, supporting her chin and stroking under her jaw trains drinking. c, Wait for the child to remove food from the spoon held below her mouth. Keep her head and shoulders well forward as she takes the food.

Practical suggestions (Fig. 7.4)

1 Unhurried feeding period, try to make it as social and as pleasant as possible. (Do not use mealtimes in any punishment.) Speech and babbling is often socially and physically stimulated during meals as articulators are beeing exercised in feeding.

2 Feed child in his own chair as soon as possible. See feeding positions above.

3 Gently press chest and bring head well forward during feeding and swallowing.

6 Wean child from liquids to tolerate various textures, tastes through semi-solids to solids. Semi-solids may be custard, puddings, stewed fruit, egg yolk in milk, yogourt, minces etc. and introduce a solid in part of the meal, e.g., apple, rusk, long sliver of meat and hold end, pulling against the food, so that the child bites off a piece.

7 Tip child forward and down if he gags and chokes at first and maintain calmness. Do not bang him on his back.

8 Correct one thing at a time, never scold; praise child's independent achievements.

9 Ignore messing and remember this is a normal process of acquiring self-feeding. Teach him to wipe his mouth and wipe the table top. A newspaper should protect the floor.

10 Support under the child's chin for drinking or to help taking food and closing the mouth. Also stroke under chin to stimulate swallowing. Fingers may have to be held under and above the lips to stimulate mouth closure and chewing. Chewing can also be helped by manipulating the child's cheek muscles. Lips must be closed.

11 Place a little on the spoon at a time, wait for the child to use his lips to take the food. Offer the spoon from in front of the child's mouth and below him and do *not* scrape the food and spoon off the top of his teeth and gums.

12 Aids: non-slip mat for bowls; stable bowls or bowl with edge; cup or beaker with rim; weighted bottoms on cups, or fix into suction or sponge rubber if needed; two handles are easier than one and make him use both hands; never use a spout or edge for drinking which leads to sucking; only use straws much later to exercise mouth closure but not to train drinking. Spoons should be unbreakable plastic, shallow, large or small according to each child. A long handled spoon makes it possible for both child and adult to hold the spoon simultaneously for guided feeding. Use angled spoons and special adaptations in much older children.

Handles of utensils may be thickened with rubberzote, clay and other materials.

Note Speech therapists and occupational therapists will advise on feeding and special problems should be referred to them.

Development of dressing—brief summary.

6–12 months   Child is supported in sitting, during dressing.

10–12 months   Child may put out arm or leg for dressing and cooperate in other ways.

15 months   Take off shoes, hat.

18 months   Take off gloves, socks, unzip.

2 years   Take off pants. Put on shoes, hat, but unable to replace pants.

3 years   Take off all clothes. Confusion of back and front, right and left, two legs in one hole of trousers etc.

4–5 years   Dresses self, becomes careless about details, such as tucking in shirt etc. All buttons, laces, ties not possible until 6 years.

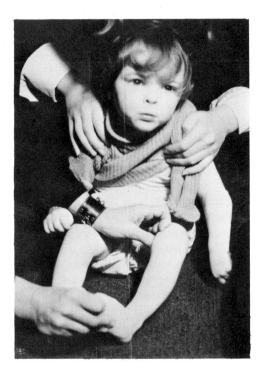

Fig. 7.5   The child is held flexed for dressing and play. Tailor-sitting is being obtained. Press beneath the big toe and bend hip and knee outward in order to overcome excessive leg extension-adduction for, say, a nappy change, sock removal and getting her into tailor-sitting.

Practical suggestions

1   Development varies greatly and too much must not be expected of the child. Dressing however is important for training perception, balance, movements, and as a source for speech and language development.

2   Begin any dressing activity for the child but let him finish it himself. If he can carry it all out himself, give him time and do not hurriedly do it for him if he is struggling on his own.

3 Vary positions for dressing to discover the easiest one for the child.

4 Dress and undress for bathing, swimming and other purposes but not for 'exercise'.

5 Type of clothing: loose fitting garments, large sleeves and arm holes (raglan) elastic necks and waistbands, large buttons, zips with knobs, velcro fastenings are required. Non-slippery materials are preferable to nylon. Tabs on front or top of shirts and dresses and back of boots are useful to guide the child. Avoid laces and small fastenings.

6 Put the more affected arm in first. Try putting both arms in first then pull dress or jumper over the head.

Note Occupational therapists will advise on dressing techniques and clothing ideas.

Development of play—brief outline.

This is the development of *learning through play*. This is closely correlated with the development of hand function and the development of intersensory relationships and perception.

> *0–6 months* Visual fixation and pursuit, hand-eye coordination and bring hands to midline and grasp, drop, reach and grasp, touch etc. Play with parts of body, mothers face, nearby materials. Amuses self for short intervals.
>
> *6–12 months* Rolling, crawling, supported cruising and other gross motor activities to explore, strengthen body generally and enjoy moving. Hand function development using toys or objects. Investigates and experiments with increasing energy.
>
> *12 months–2 years* Solitary play but imitates another child or adult. Uses large equipment, swings, balls, toys on wheels to push and pull. Sand and water play. Enjoys small objects such as shells, pebbles, buttons—often taken to mouth until 15 months of age.
>
> *2–3 years* Rough and tumble play. As above only with more perceptual and conceptual ideas. Begins imaginative play ('Let's pretend'). Solitary and parallel play.
>
> *3–4 years* Plays with other children. Imaginative play, dressing up. As above but not as energetic.
>
> *6 years* Games with rules, arts and crafts. 'Tricks'.

Practical suggestions

1 Play differs at different ages, but it is impossible to have it strictly classified as the child's personality, opportunities and intelligence affect this. Social and cultural backgrounds also affect play.

2 Play is usually a synonym for exploration and experimentation and is a serious affair for the child. Play can also be relaxing, working out emotions, imitating reality in order to understand it in imaginative play, and obtaining satisfactions and development of the child's personality. It is often messy, dirty, untidy and destructive as well as creative and constructive, in the adult sense.

3 Show the child how to use a toy, but wherever possible see if he can find things out for himself.

4 Do not interfere with any child who is concentrating on a play activity unless absolutely essential.

Technique's for carrying the child correctly are given in Figs. 7.6–7.11:

1 To stimulate head control.

2 To correct any abnormal postures.

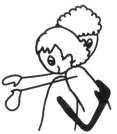

Fig. 7.6 Both the arms are over the adult's shoulder for symmetry, straighten back and raise head. Keep the legs apart, and hips flat if necessary in spastics. Bring tight arms away from their habitual positions next to the child.

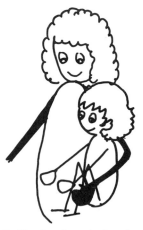

Fig. 7.7 For head control and correcting an excessively extended child, help bring hands down and together helps control an athetoid or floppy child.

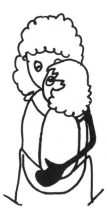

Fig. 7.8 Use of both arms, eye-to-eye contact, separate tightly adducted legs or very extended legs. Move the child to points around the adult's hips to find the most corrective posture of legs for him.

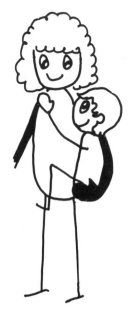

Fig. 7.9   Use of both arms, eye-to-eye contact, separate tightly adducted legs or very extended legs. Move the child to points around the adult's hips to find the most corrective posture of legs for him.

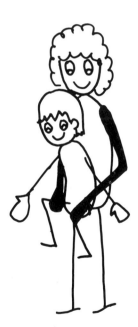
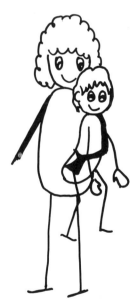

Fig. 7.10   Head and trunk control, if the child is moved slightly away from the adult's chest. Correct extended-adducted-internally rotated legs of a spastic (for child who holds his legs tightly straight, pressed together and turned inward).

Fig. 7.11   Stimulates greater hand and trunk control for floppy and other children. Hold child at chest and under his armpits and/or under his buttocks as well.

PROBLEMS OF DEFORMITY

A deformity is an abnormal position of a joint. In cerebral palsy and other developmentally delayed children abnormal joint positions rarely appear or depend on only one joint and the total child must be examined.

The deformity may be mobile or 'unfixed', which means that passive or active correction can take place. The deformity may have become 'fixed' or a contracture when there is adaptive shortening of the soft tissues or bony changes. The therapist tries to prevent deformities developing as unfixed or fixed deformities. If unfixed deformities have already appeared they are treated, but little can be done for fixed deformities. Orthopaedic surgery is indicated for fixed deformities. However, in selected cases, orthopaedic surgery is also required for unfixed deformities.

Prevention and correction of deformities in therapy and daily care should consider the causes of the deformities. However, many different causes are suggested by various authorities. The greatest difference of opinion may occur between orthopaedics and neurology. It is, however, possible for the therapist to combine many if not all viewpoints, as outlined in this chapter. The therapist may be able to classify the causes of deformity under the following headings. Some of these causes are interwoven and their relationships are discussed.

1 Immobility—total or partial.
2 Hypotonicity.
3 Hypertonicity.
4 Weakness—general or specific.
5 Abnormal reflex activity.
6 Asymmetry.
7 Involuntary movements in one repetitive pattern.
8 Growth factors.
9 Biomechanics.

Immobility—General

A general immobility of the child may be due to:

Physical handicap of hypotonicity, hypertonicity, weakness, involuntary movements and severe spasms, abnormal reflex activity (see below). Severe deformities may have already developed and these prevent further movement. The deformities themselves may then become worse and also produce others.

Other causes such as sensory loss mainly blindness, severe perceptual-motor defects, especially those related to space and body image, emotional problems, especially if the child is fearful or withdrawn, mental subnormality, social deprivation and malnutrition. Most of these reasons tend to create lethargic unmotivated children, who prefer to be immobile.

When many of the above causes combine in the same child, deformities are likely to occur.

Immobility—Partial

Despite some or many of the above causes a child may acquire a few similar postures and a few stereotyped movements. This is well-known in spastic and severely mentally subnormal children, and is particularly dangerous for them. The few postures and movements which spastics or tension athetoids prefer are usually abnormal in pattern. The repetition of these postures and movements leads to deformity into these joint positions.

Hypotonicity

The floppy baby may be due to many neurological causes affecting the muscles themselves, their spinal connections or the central nervous system. Therefore hypotonic babies and children, whether they are cerebral palsied or have any of the myopathies, infantile muscular dystrophies or other conditions, all present the common problem of immobility. They may be left lying for long periods in one or two positions, which can create deformities. For example, the 'frog position' of the legs in prone, supine or with the child propped up on pillows, or in the half slumped sitting position against the pillows or in a pram, may all lead to deformities in the legs, especially in the hips.

As discussed on page 40 the common characteristic of most floppy babies is the absence of all or some of the normal postural mechanisms. The neck, trunk, shoulder and pelvic girdle muscles are not being activated by these mechanisms, and appear weak and hypotonic. Hypotonia is not always associated with total weakness. Fair or even good voluntary movement may be present, but it is not enough to make the child mobile. He needs a background of postural reactions, i.e. automatic postural muscle action. Without this he cannot get out of the few positions in which he is left during the day and night.

Some hypotonic children may develop some of the postural mechanisms and develop to sitting and standing. However, they carry out these levels of development in an abnormal way. Common abnormal patterns which can lead to deformity are round backs, scoliosis, lordosis and hip flexion, hyperextended knees ('back-knees'), valgus knees ('knock-knees') and valgus feet (flat feet). One or all of these postures may be present in the hypotonic child.

Hypertonicity

This is the most important cause of deformity. The creation of the deformities are, however, not dependent on the hypertonicity as such. There are five main aspects responsible for deformities in hypertonic (spastic or rigid) children, as well as the immobility already mentioned.

1 Hypertonicity.
2 Abnormal reflex activity.
3 'Weak' antagonists.
4 Specific inefficiency of spastic muscles.
5 Co-contraction (abnormal).

Hypertonicity Hypertonic muscle groups tend to pull the joints into abnormal positions. In the baby and young child these abnormal positions can be anticipated by the tendency of the child to prefer certain postures and movements, and by the examination of the muscles using sudden passive stretch. There is an abnormal reaction to this sudden stretch, given by the examiner of the hypertonic muscles. It is either a 'clasp-knife' spastic reaction of a 'lead pipe' or 'cogwheel' rigid reaction. The tendency of hypertonic muscles is to shorten, which will cause *one aspect* of the deformity. In the baby this muscle shortening appears in abnormal postures threatening deformity, and in time these abnormal postures become habitual and can be clearly observed. If left still longer they become fixed abnormal positions or contractures.

Hypertonic muscles pull the joints into patterns of abnormal postures of the whole child or at least of the whole limb. However one joint may be more deformed than the others within the pattern. It is important to CHECK EACH JOINT as well as observe the PATTERN OF ABNORMAL POSTURE and movement. In this way both the neurological and orthopaedic pictures should be combined (see Table 5.1, p. 51).

Hypertonicity may pull the joints into abnormal positions at rest. Hypertonicity may be *absent at rest* but only elicited on passive stretch. When elicited on passive stretch, hypertonicity may still *not* produce abnormal positions in function. Hypertonicity may be absent at rest, minimal on passive stretch but only be obvious on *weight bearing* and during function. Finally, hypertonicity may create abnormal positions at rest, show very hyperactive stretch reflexes on passive stretch and also show the same abnormal, shortened positions in function.

The therapist and especially those involved in daily care should treat the hypertonicity which appears *in function*, as seen in the developmental motor skills. See especially Abnormal Postures in Sitting (pp. 114–117), Abnormal Postures in Standing (pp. 139–147).

Abnormal reflex activity This is another aspect of hypertonicity which is discussed below.

The 'weak' antagonists to the spastic muscle groups Sharrard states that spasticity alone does not create deformity. It is the muscle imbalance between the spastic muscles and their weak antagonists, which leads to deformity. The antagonists of the spastic muscle groups are working at a mechanical disadvantage to the tight pull of spastic muscle groups. They cannot counter the pull of the spastic muscles and appear too weak to do so. In time they really become weak from disuse. It is necessary to treat this muscle imbalance by reducing the spasticity and strengthening the antagonists.

Although many orthopaedic surgeons talk of the muscle imbalance, they unfortunately say that the spastic muscles are *strong* and the antagonists are *weak*. This is rarely so in every case. It is the strong *pull* of the still spastic muscle that is strong, and not the spastic muscle work itself. Unless this is recognised, postoperative physiotherapy as well as therapy of hypertonic children without operation will be inadequate.

Specific inefficiency of hypertonic especially spastic muscles Spastic muscles are not paralysed muscles. They can contract. However, they are often *not* strong muscles. Spasm or spasticity must not be confused with strong and efficient muscle action.

Once spasticity is decreased, spastic muscles may reveal great weakness. Also spastic muscles may be able to act in only one part of their range and not in the rest of the range (Plum). They act better in one part of the range than in another part (Knott). Cotton emphasises how children with, say, flexor spasticity of the hips cannot actively flex their hips in order to reach their feet. The limited range of motion in spastic muscles may be due to their inelasticity or weakness or both (Tardieu & Tabary). The electromyograph of the type of muscle contraction in spastic muscles has been shown as abnormal (Holt) [33, 44, 66, 36, 20].

It may be that this inefficiency of action of the spastic muscles may contribute to deformity. Their action as well as their tightness should not be ignored during the therapeutic regime for the prevention and correction of deformity. Motor activities should not only strengthen or facilitate or activate the apparently weak antagonists of abnormal postures held by stiff spastic muscles, but also activate the spastic muscles themselves *in their full range.*

Abnormal co-contraction and abnormal synergies The abnormal tightness of the hypertonic muscle means they do not 'let go' during movement. This type of incoordination can be called abnormal co-contraction. The hypertonic muscle co-contracts with its antagonist's action. This hampers the efforts made by the antagonists against the pull of the hypertonic muscles and enhances the creation of deformity. Abnormal 'neurological organisation' or 'abnormal synergies' or 'abnormal patterning' are all similar terms meaning that there is a recurring abnormal performance in hypertonic children, which tends to lead to deformity within those un-desirable patterns. This is the same aspect discussed under Partial Immo-bility. An example of this occurs in the use of abnormal reflexes discussed below.

Weakness—General and Specific

This heading is only given, as so many workers in cerebral palsy use this term. It should, however, be more clearly defined.

General weakness has already been discussed under hypotonicity and general immobility. The absence of the postural reflex mechanism creates general weakness.

Specific weakness has been discussed as the weakness of the antagonists in hypertonicity, the weakness of the spastic muscles themselves and under asymmetry the weakness due to absence of a specific postural mechanism on one side. With any partial immobility specific rather than general weak-ness will be the weakness usually observed.

Weakness may be present in voluntary contraction or not on specific voluntary contraction but only during the more complex situation of var-ious motor functions.

Weakness may be present on voluntary contraction of a specific muscle group. On the other hand that specific muscle may act well on voluntary contraction but appear weak when used within a motor function or motor developmental skill. Both may occur.

Abnormal reflex activity (see pp. 55–59)

This may be persisting primitive reflex reactions or pathological reflex reactions. It is not the reflex *as such*, but the recurring stimulation of the reflex by adults or by the child in his own efforts to move, which may lead to deformity. However not all hypertonic children resort to use of abnormal reflexes to move.

Examples:

Opisthotonus or repeated extensor thrusts in the legs only, tends to lead to a fixed extensor posture.

Asymmetrical tonic neck reactions or any other asymmetrical limb postures created by head turning may lead to deformities in the limbs, a scoliosis and/or a torticollis. Extensor postures are associated with asymmetrical tonic neck reactions.

Symmetrical tonic neck reflexes may occur in severe cases. Immobility and lack of treatment may lead to deformities within these patterns.

Reflex stepping may aggravate hypertonic plantarflexors, adductors and extensors if this reflex is used to 'walk' the child frequently.

Excessive supporting reaction may be overstimulated by, say, 'baby bouncers' and increases the deformities of the legs, especially equinus and extensor-adductor postures.

Excessive suspension or 'lift reaction' [36]   If the child is lifted or suspended under the armpits and lowered to the ground, and there is an excessive plantarflexion [36], Tardieu suggests this may cause equinus.

Active use of total flexion reactions, withdrawal reflexes in kicking, during rolling, crawling, kneeling. The withdrawal reaction which combines hip-knee and ankle flexion rather than hip-flexion-knee *extension* and ankle flexion may be used in (heel strike) stepping. This hip and knee flexion instead of hip extension-knee flexion or other such synergia may be used in swing-through or 'push-off' in gait. The repeated use of flexion in all these movements or postures tends to flexion deformity.

Use of total extension reflexes as in using the extensor thrust in active kicking, when bounced on the feet in standing, during rolling and creeping along the floor, may lead to deformities into these patterns of extension.

Asymmetry

1   Asymmetrical distribution of hypertonus.
2   Asymmetrical development of postural reactions.
3   Asymmetrical presence or persistence of abnormal reflex.
4   Asymmetrical growth of legs. See abnormal postures and asymmetry in Development of Standing (p. 141), Sitting (p. 117) and Prone development (p. 87).

Involuntary movement in one repetitive pattern.

Any repeated flexor spasms or involuntary athetoid 'kicking' with hip and/or knee flexion, or 'pawing' an athetoid leg may give rise to tightness in knees or hips and knee joints. Similarly and less commonly extensor spasms or rotary involuntary movement may create tightness.

Growth factors [36, 37, 84]

There are four main factors which cause or aggravate the development of deformity.

1 The difference in leg length, see Asymmetry in Abnormal Postures in Standing. (Difference in arm length is not related to the genesis of deformation.)

2 Spurts of growth in cerebral palsied children and adolescents are linked with deterioration and increase of deformities. The unequal growth of bone and muscle, increase in height and especially increase in weight seem to bring on deformities. Usually there would also be less mobility as older children need to spend longer hours at their studies.

3 The mechanism of growth and spasticity have been studied by Sharrard and by Tardieu and Tabary. Sharrard believes it is the stronger spastic muscles imbalanced with their weaker antagonists, which pull unevenly on growing bones and create deformity. Tabary *et al.* showed that the shortened spastic muscles have a diminution of sarcomeres compared with normally mobile and extensible muscles. The immobile, inelastic, shortened spastic muscles grow abnormally in relation to bone and deformities increase with growth. Orthopaedic surgery is inevitable in their view [37].

4 The specific bony structure of the hip in spastic children does not change as it normally would with growth, due to spasticity and non-weight bearing. The neck of the femur remains in anteversion and the shaft/neck angle of valgus does not decrease. This is part of the reason for hip deformity, and dislocations.

Biomechanics

Every joint should be considered in the treatment of deformities whether with or without orthopaedic surgery. This is due to the biomechanics of deformity. These are not only dependent on the spastic muscle groups, each of which may flex one joint and extend another, e.g. hamstrings, rectus, gastrocnemius, and their relationship to weakness or on the effect on other joints or in the biomechanics of spasticity (page 142). The more important clue, is the presence or absence of the postural mechanisms of postural fixation, counterpoising and the locomotive reflexes which initiate the step and lateral sway. When these are abnormal the child compensates by using abnormal postures in order to maintain balance in functions such as sitting, standing, crawling and walking. See Development of Sitting and Standing, pp. 111–146. Occasionally hip flexion deformity or equinus deformity may disbalance the child, but it is usual the disbalance *of the child* which increases hip flexion in compensation for falling backward.

Therapy and daily care

Treatment aims based on the causes of deformity discussed are therefore:

1 Motivation of movement throughout the day. However, movements must be varied and where possible of normal pattern.

2 Frequent changes of the child's posture.

3 Postures and movements must include:

Passive elongation of hypertonic muscles and soft tissues.

Active and full range of movement of antagonists to hypertonic muscles.

Active and full range of movement of hypertonic muscles including active work in their elongated position.

4 Correct any asymmetries of posture, movement or balance.

5 Train the normal postural mechanisms and locomotor reactions.

6 Control recurring involuntary motion in one pattern.

7 Counteract any relevant pathological reflexes.

8 Treat the biomechanics of deformity and not just deformity in one joint.

As in the discussion of the causes many of the aims interact with each other.

Techniques

Techniques for all the aims mentioned above are presented in the Chapter 6 on Developmental Training. There are, however, additional methods which may be required for individual children. These will be offered *with a summary of some of those already mentioned* in the book. It may be helpful to discuss each joint separately, in case one joint is threatening to deform or is already showing more deformity than the others within the total patterns of function. The orthopaedic surgeon usually studies the child for the major deforming factor. In summarising the methods it may be helpful to remember the following points in connection with the Aims of Therapy.

Elongation of hypertonic muscles takes place in positioning the child in equipment, in splints, corrective moulds and braces, in plaster of Paris, in orthopaedic surgery. Elongation is made possible by any techniques which reduce hypertonus. Active work of the antagonists to the shortened muscles will also involve elongation of these shortened muscles.

Active and full range of antagonists takes place if the child activates his muscles to hold any of the 'positioning' rather than only depend on therapist's hands, equipment, bracing or plasters to hold lengthened position of hypertonic muscles or shortened muscles.

Some workers (Rood) suggest that there is a reciprocal relaxation of shortened muscles when there is activation of their antagonists. Movements which correct abnormal postures are movements which activate antagonists to the shortened or spastic muscles. They are strengthened and their 'disuse' weakness treated in such movement [28, 35].

Active and full range of hypertonic muscles in movements as well as the above, also help to mobilise joints and prevent or counteract deformity.

Reduce Hypertonicity In order to obtain the aims of therapy above, especially in relation to the elongation of hypertonic muscles and make it easier to activate their antagonists, it is important to reduce the hypertonicity. A reduction or inhibition of hypertonicity also helps to obtain more efficient muscle action in the hypertonic muscle groups themselves. Reduction of hypertonicity includes the following techniques:

1 Use of rotation in movements.
2 Use of gentle prolonged stretch in passive movements, equipment, plasters or splintage.
3 Activation of antagonists on their own or with other methods, may inhibit the spastic agonists.
4 Ice treatments.
5 Medical treatments using drugs, localised procaine blocks, alcohol (phenol) injections. Neurectomies are rarely used to cut off nerve supply to spastic muscles, as this also cuts off their ability to work as well.
6 Vibration techniques (Hagbarth & Eklund, Rood) [82, 53].
7 Repeated contractions of spastic muscles to obtain autoinhibition (Rood). An active contraction of the antagonists must follow immediately.

SUMMARY

THE HIP DEFORMITIES

Hip flexion-adduction-internal rotation One component may be greater than the others. The shape of the hip joint may be abnormal e.g. the acetabulum is shallow, neck of femur anteverted; subdislocation and dislocation may occur.

Therapy and daily care

Positioning Prone lying, legs apart on conical-shaped pommel, in prone wedges, prone board; standing boards, standing frames, standing tables, sitting with legs apart, externally rotated, side-sitting, tailor-sitting, sitting in chairs with pommels; stand or sit straddling equipment or rolls; carrying with legs apart and turned out over adult's hip or over adult shoulder pressing child's hip flat with legs apart.

Splintage and bracing Abduction pants used in all positions; abduction splint (Grenier) used in standing and walking; long leg braces with pelvic band; rotation coil attached to pelvic band and shoe for external rotation, (but check for any abnormal effect of tibial torsion), 'twisters' (Fig. 6.162) for milder spastics [94].

Plaster of Paris   Long leg spicas to incorporate hip extension-abduction rarely work. Excessive flexor spasms usually occur after removal of plaster.

Ice treatment to reduce hypertonicity.
1   Apply towels wrung out in chopped ice and water to adductor surface of leg for 3–4 minutes. In addition place the child in tailor-sitting or over a roll *while* the ice pack is tied onto his thighs. Repeat applications of ice packs. Carry out active abduction movements as well.
2   Wring rough towels out in ice so that ice flakes cling to the towelling. Roll the whole leg from groin to feet in the towel for 3–4 minutes. Carry out leg patterns with rotation in the hip during and after ice application as well as positioning. Repeat.

Active exercise to antagonists
1   See Developmental Training for active hip extension, hip abduction, hip external rotation in creeping, rolling from prone to supine, active extension in 'standing tall', in stand and reach overhead. Counterpoising techniques using leg extension, abduction, external rotation (Figs. 6.37, 6.38, 6.158 in four point kneeling and in standing, squatting or sitting rise to standing, kneeling rise to standing, four foot kneeling rise to upright standing, and other postural changes.
2   Other examples are given in Figs. 8.1–8.10. Emphasise the movement of the antagonists to the deformity e.g. the extensors in flexion deformities.

Active exercise to agonists and antagonists   See Developmental Training of creeping (flexion and extension of legs) (p. 79) counterpoising techniques in crawling positions (p. 88) and standing position (p. 155). Sitting, touch floor and raise up in standing, see Figs. 8.1–8.10.

Orthopaedic surgery for hip deformities may be: Iliopsoas elongation, adductor tenotomies, obturator neurectomies, rotation osteotomies; for hip dislocation-adductor tenotomy and obturator neurectomies or rotation osteotomy or removal of head of femur. Surgeons recommend early weight bearing and abduction *with* extension to prevent subdislocation of the hips in cerebral palsy.

Hip extension deformity

Therapy and daily care

Positioning   Chairs to increase flexion, and overcoming (p. 123) extension in standing and walking training, and correct carrying in flexion positions (p. 205). Use heel-sitting, squatting and crook-sitting.

Splintage and bracing, plasters, ice not used as positioning seems to be simplest and more effective.

Active movements of flexion and of flexion and extension, see Developmental training of creeping (p. 77), crawling (p. 86) and standing (p. 159). See Figs. 8.1–8.10.

Note To overcome excessive extension of head, trunk and hips and knees manually and in equipment, it is important to flex the child at his head and shoulders *and* at his hip joint. Hold his head and shoulders, hold under his knees and flex him 'into a ball'. His extensor spasm, thrust or constant extensor hypertonus decreases in this position.
Orthopaedic surgery is not used.

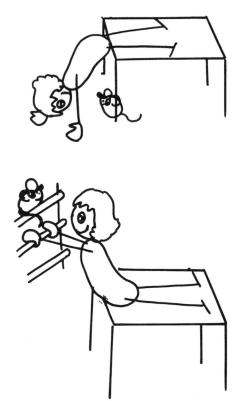

Fig. 8.1 Bend over edge of mother's lap, large ball or couch, raise up and bend down again. Hold rungs and 'walk up' for level hip extension. Keep legs apart and turned out if necessary. Child raises head and trunk up in association with hip extension. Initial support may be given by your hand on his chest. Avoid abnormal extensor thrust.

Fig. 8.2 Child's legs over mother's lap, edge of bed large ball, or roll. Bring legs down to floor (hip flexion) into bed (hip extension). Hold knees and thighs apart in external rotation to encourage hip extension-abduction-external rotation if required. Raise *one* leg at a time to control lordosis (Fig. 8.6). Child may grasp side of table or both his arms are held elevated-abducted and externally rotated by adult if abnormal flexion in arm and trunk is present.

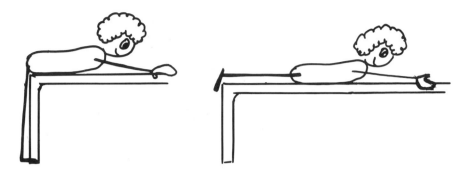

Fig. 8.3 Legs of child held in abduction-external rotation. Active raise of child's hips into extension. *Avoid* use of lordosis to do this. Legs may be on lap of therapist, on low stool or with his feet flat on the ground for 'bridging' the pelvis into extension. Manual resistance may be given to anterior superior iliac spines to augment extension. Obtain flexion by asking child to bend knees to chest then repeat above extension activity.

Fig. 8.4 The child actively stretches down and comes up to sitting with or without grasping your hands. For babies you may use the large ball, or roll. The child may also bend sideways to the floor for scoliosis (to side of the covexity).

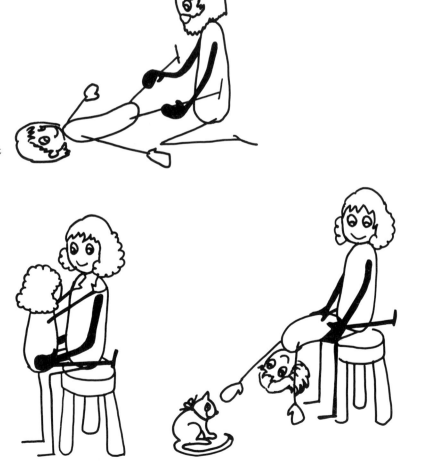

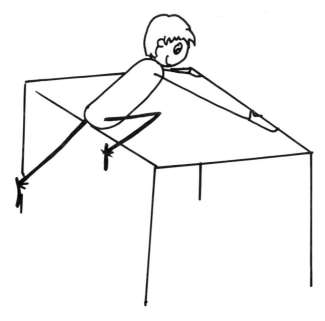

Fig. 8.5 One knee held bent to chest during hip extension of the other leg, to counteract lordosis. Carry this out in side-lying or in prone. Also flex-abduct-externally rotate extended leg for action of those agonists.

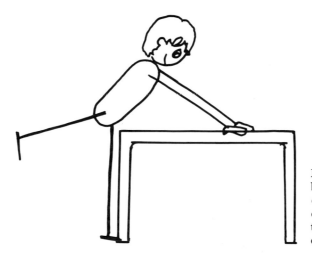

Fig. 8.6 Child leans forward onto ball, table, roll, during active hip extension of each leg. Lordosis is more easily controlled this way. Next, flex the leg so that foot reaches highbar or even table.

KNEE DEFORMITIES

Knee flexion
Therapy and daily care

Positioning   Prone-lying with straight knees, sitting with straight knees on the floor, in floor-seat or sit on a low chair if back rounds in sitting. Use knee gaiters in sitting and in standing.

Splintage and bracing   Knee gaiters, long leg calipers, knee splints.

Plasters from hip to ankle are useful ('stove pipe plasters').

Ice treatment to whole leg (see Hip flexion above).

Active movements for knee extensors and for knee flexors and extensors. See Developmental Training for Hip, see Figs. 8.1–8.10.

Orthopaedic Surgery   Various operations on the hamstrings, such as partial hamstring tenotomy or hamstring slide (Eggers), hamstring transplant e.g. lengthen semitendinosis, transpose semimembrinosus and detach gracilis.

Knee hyperextension
Therapy and daily care

Positioning   Keep child off his feet sometimes, use sitting on chair, side-sit, tailor-sitting, kneel-sitting, crook-sitting. If child is standing already, stand with knee pieces preventing hyperextension; use shoes with higher heel to throw child's weight into knee flexion posture, *if* his plantarflexors are not shortened (see Standing, Fig. 6.164).

Splintage and bracing   Knee pieces which lock with knee in midline, but allow knee flexion motion. Not necessary in many children.

Plasters and ice treatment for plantarflexors of the feet, if this is the cause of hyperextended knees, or for hamstrings.

Passive stretch and movement   Hyperextension may be due to tight plantarflexors. Passive stretch of these muscles is indicated.

Active movement of knee flexors, but more important dorsiflexors of ankles if tight plantarflexors are present.

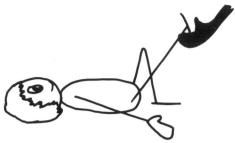

Fig. 8.7   One knee flexed to chest or flexed with foot flat. Press other leg into extension into adult's hand, sponge rubber surface, soft couch. Child's hips raise into extension with his weight on one foot. Full flexion of each hip should be carried out actively if required. Arms straight, and hands pressed flat or grasping edge of bed.

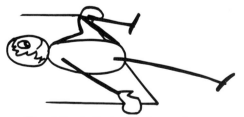

Fig. 8.8 *Activate agonists and antagonists* and full range of active hip and knee motion. Use of arm extension is incorporated in these exercises.

Fig. 8.9 *Activate agonists and antagonists* and full range of active hip and knee motion. Use of arm extension is incorporated in these exercises.

Active work for fixation of pelvis, which is often the cause of hyperextended knees. See Crawling Development (p. 86), Standing Development (p. 160) and use of 'bear-walk' in Prone Development (p. 91).

Orthopaedic surgery: hyperextended knees are secondary to plantarflexor deformity or hip flexion deformity these joints may sometimes require surgery.

DEFORMITY OF THE FEET

Equinus and Equino-varus

Therapy and daily care

Positioning   Prone lying with feet over edge of wedge or pillows, prone boards with heels down; sitting in chairs with heels flat on ground; stand-

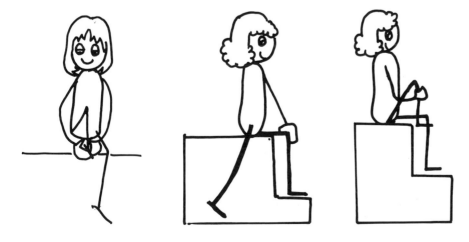

Fig. 8.10 *Activate agonists and antagonists* and full range of active hip and knee motion. Use of arm extension is incorporated in these exercises.

ing feet held flat on ground; standing in boots with raised soles; stand facing up on inclined platform; 'bear-walk' positions.

Splintage and bracing   Below-knee irons with backstop, boots with raise on soles. Strap to keep the child's heel down in his boot. The strap should be wider and padded as it crosses the front of his ankle.

Plasters   Technique described below (Fig. 8.15).

Ice treatment to whole leg or the ice pack to plantarflexors only.

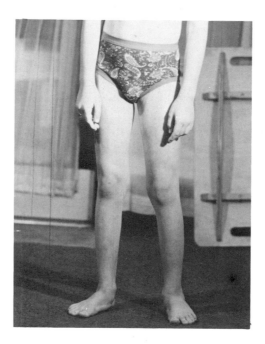

Fig. 8.11   Child with valgus feet.

Passive stretch and movement   Hold the knee flexed with one hand, and grasp the heel and foot with your other hand. Gently dorsiflex foot as far as possible. Hold in dorsiflexion as you passively extend the child's knee.

Do not evert the child's foot as you push it up into dorsiflexion. Stretch must be slow and maintained. Ask child to hold foot up in dorsiflexion with you.

Other suggestions for *Passive stretch*, including active dorsiflexions:
1   Child stands and leans forward to wall to stretch heel cords.
2   With child's legs apart, turned out, push both his feet into dorsiflexion.

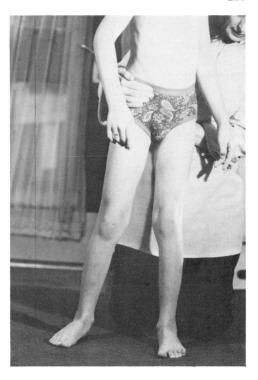

Fig. 8.12 Rotate pelvis to stimulate action of foot muscles to correct valgus. Rotate against your manual resistance at the hip in front and behind.

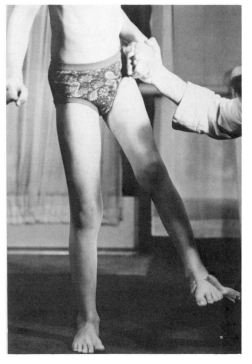

Fig. 8.13 Stand, tip the child onto outside of his foot to provoke action of foot muscles to correct valgus. Child may move his pelvis laterally against your hand to obtain inversion of feet, backwards for dorsiflexion, forwards for plantarflexion.

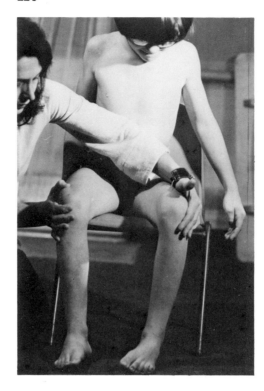

Fig. 8.14 Correction of abnormal adduction, internal rotation or valgus feet. Press his knees outward against your hands or the therapist turns his knees outwards for him. This may be done in sitting, in standing or in squatting positions.

3 Stand and lunge forward; Half-kneeling lunge forward on front foot.

4 Sitting heels on small inclined foot board obtaining dorsiflexion; Stand with heels down, child facing up, on inclined board.

5 Bear walk with heels down (Fig. 6.164, 9–12 months level).

6 Standing on tipping board or rocker, slowly tipped back with child's heels held down (Figs. 6.155, 6.174).

7 Walk on heels if possible. Raise the soles of his shoes, or remove heels off his shoes.

8 See Figs. 8.2, 8.6, 8.7, 8.10.

9 Always sit in a chair with heels down.

Active dorsiflexion

1 Hold the young baby's ankles, lift them up and slowly suspend the child upside down. Reflex dorsiflexion may occur.

2 'Reflex creeping' stimulates dorsiflexion. Other leg flexion patterns may do this (Fig. 6.39; pp. 79, 88, 155).

3 Brushing, quick icing to dorsiflexors following passive stretch or ice to plantarflexors.

4 'Bone-pounding' or striking heel of foot on surface stimulates dorsiflexion.

5 Use of tipping board or tip child back into his heels may stimulate dorsi-flexion of his feet (Fig. 6.174).

6 Walk up inclined plane.

7 Draw faces on child's feet, and ask him to dorsiflex or raise his feet to look at the face, or to touch a toy and so on.

8 Child to practise heel strike in walking.

9 Use pattern of hip flexion-adduction external rotation, knee extension, foot dorsiflexion, with child in sitting over edge of bed or in supported standing. Use stretch, touch, pressure and resistance if this method (P.N.F.) is known (Fig. 6.158 b).

Orthopaedic surgery Surgeon may carry out lengthening of Achilles tendon (z-plasty) or gastrocnemius slide, e.g. volpius operation.

Valgus feet (pronated)

Positioning Have hips and knees turned out during sitting, round sit on the floor feet in varus, hips externally rotated. Correct equinus if present as valgus is often overcompensation for this.

Splintage and bracing Correct shoes or boots with inside raise, inside the shoe or outside on the sole or both; use moulded foot support to inner side of feet; below-knee iron with inside T-strap; flare the heel or sole on the inner side so that it juts out slightly at the base [95].

Ice treatment Occasionally may be used for spastic plantarflexion and for spastic peroneii.

Plasters See below.

Passive stretch as for equinus but include some inversion.

Activity As for equinus, but emphasise inversion. Figs. 8.11, 8.12, 8.13, 8.14. Tap the Bone at the heel and malleolii on one side to provoke inversion.

Orthopaedic Surgery If secondary to other deformities. Severely deformed feet may also be treated with Grice's operation to the joints (Triple arthrodesis).

Varus feet

See Equinus for treatment and Figs. 8.12–8.14; tap bone at heel and malleoli all to provoke eversion. Plasters, splintage and bracing are used with adjustment to the opposite side to that used for valgus.

Clenched toes or everted toes

This disappears with correct weight bearing and balance training. Heel must be on the ground and equinus treated. 'Flick' toes up as child takes weight. Use sponge or felt to hold toes corrected while balance develops. Excessive toe flexion occurs if standing is too early for the child.

ARM DEFORMITY

Shoulder flexion-adduction-internal rotation

Positioning   Elevation of arms on high table, over rolls. Hold the child's upper arms and turn them out (Figs. 6.25, 6.105). Hold this position during play (Fig. 7.3, p. 196).

Splintage, bracing, plasters   These are not used.
Occasionally a 'figure 8 scarf' to hold his shoulders back is helpful.

Ice treatment of the whole arm.

Passive stretch and activity   In positioning and during activities. See Developmental training of creeping (p. 86), crawling (p. 86) and counterpoising (p. 87), sitting and counterpoising with arm elevation (Figs. 6.177, 6.182), arms over large ball during training of standing (p. 150), arm elevation in standing and counterpoising (p. 154). Correct *shoulder retraction* in Developmental training.

Orthopaedic surgery   Not commonly used.

Elbow flexion

Positioning   See 'Shoulder' and how to keep elbow straight in all Developmental training and Chapter 7.

Splintage   Elbow corsets.

Passive stretch   NONE as this is dangerous.

Active movements and correction of posture see Sitting (Fig. 6.105), Arms (p. 173).

Ice treatment of the whole arm.

Orthopaedic surgery   Rare.

Wrist flexion and ulnar deviation

See Developmental Training and Hand Function (pp. 169–198).

Orthopaedic surgery Occasionally to wrist flexors, or stabilisation of the wrist joint.

HAND AND THUMB DEFORMITIES (pp. 178–180, see Appendix)

DEFORMITIES OF TRUNK AND HEAD

See Figs. 8.1–8.10 [96].
   See Developmental Training, especially in Sitting (p. 114) and Standing (p. 139). See Chairs (p. 123). Prone boards (Fig. 6.149). Some orthopaedic surgeons recommend braces for scoliosis and some operate as well.

GENERAL CONSIDERATIONS RELATED TO SURGERY

The physiotherapist should help the surgeon prepare the child and his family for surgery, if that has been recommended. *Their cooperation is most important*. The child and family should understand:
1 The surgery is not a cure, but an episode in the total rehabilitation programme. The degree of drive and *sometimes* intelligence of the child affects the results of surgery.
2 There will be a setback before the ultimate progress is more obvious.
3 How to look after the child in plaster.
4 How to help with postoperative physiotherapy.
5 How to apply any splintage or braces to maintain improvement by surgery.
6 To try and maintain confidence and an encouraging atmosphere.
   It is best if the child's own physiotherapist can be the one to treat him before the operation in the hospital and follow up in the home or centre. Otherwise she and the parents should at least introduce the child to the hospital environment, meet some of the staff and generally let the child know what is going to happen there. Possible psychological disturbance due to surgery and its associated hospitalisation must not be ignored, as it has been known to affect children for years, and also hamper the physical advances gained by the surgery.

PREOPERATIVE PHYSIOTHERAPY

Hips, knees and feet

1 Train all muscle groups *not only* the antagonists to the deformity.

2 Train all *posture—balance reactions*. Results of surgery also depend on activity of these mechanisms, or as many of them as possible.

3 Measure child for any splints or braces ordered for the child's use post-operatively.

POSTOPERATIVE PHYSIOTHERAPY AND CARE

Hip and knee operations

In plaster Spicas with broomstick to hold abduction or plaster from groins to feet, with the broomstick, may follow for 6 weeks to 3 months. Some adductor tenotomies may not be followed by any plasters.

1 Check that child's head and trunk are kept in alignment. Discourage sacral sitting, holding onto the broomstick (see positions in 3).

2 Carry child over your shoulder keeping his hips flat with your hand.

3 Change position from bed to sitting on chair with board for legs, or on foot supports. Use prone as on prone board in 4, and also in standing supported, in plaster. Weight bearing in plasters is important and permission to do this must be obtained as soon as possible.

4 Use prone board on wheels with wide board for legs. Keep hips flat with a band across them. Place ankles on roll of towels, pillow under chest.

5 Plasters may be split at end of 3 weeks after Egger's operation.

6 In plaster, carry out extension movement of head, arms and back. Sleep on pillows under his side and one leg whilst he lies slightly on his other side.

Out of plaster

1 Use splintage for knees to control flexor spasms.

2 Treat pain and swelling, dry skin as for all postoperative cases.

3 Gentle movements in as much range as possible.

4 Continue balance training whenever possible and preferably in standing. Therefore place the child on his feet as soon as possible with surgeon's permission.

5 Gently obtain hip and knee flexion by sitting on increasingly lower and lower chairs, over the edge of pillows and in exercises.

6 No unrelieved sitting is to be resumed.

Foot operations

Foot operations may be followed by long leg plasters including the foot or below-knee plasters for 6 weeks.

1 Train standing as soon as possible with surgeon's permission. Walking in plaster must be emphasised. Correct pelvic-trunk alignments.

2 Extension exercises for hips and knees in all positions are required, especially in sitting rise to standing.

Out of plaster

1 Below-knee iron may be recommended by the surgeon.

2 Active dorsiflexion encouraged (see above equinus—active motion; Figs. 8.12, 8.13, 8.14).

3 Continue training postural balance mechanism in pelvis and trunk in all positions, especially standing.

4 Plantarflexion, walking on the toes and 'push off' should be trained if possible.

Use of weight bearing plasters

Indications for below-knee plaster are:

1 When child pulls up to stand on his toes only, or continues standing on toes.

2 When child stands with heels down but walks on toes.

3 When child is ready for standing and walking but cannot balance on deformed feet in either equinus, varus or equinovarus. When sitting balance is poor and feet are habitually in plantarflexion.

4 To prevent any of the above becoming fixed deformities.

5 To train a better walking pattern using the proprioceptive responses and body image of weight bearing with the heel down and the possibility of heel strike on stepping forward, made possible by the corrective plaster.

Application of plaster. Based on work by de Rijke, Culloty, Burns and Allen [113], [114].

Position   Child should lie prone with his knee bent so that dorsiflexion is easier to obtain, and to hold as the plaster is being applied.

Personnel   One person talks to the child and relaxes him and reads to him. One person applies the plaster and another person holds the foot in the corrected position. To quicken the time taken to apply the plaster an additional helper to cut and soak the plasters is needed.

Preparation of the foot and leg

1   Clean skin, apply olive oil.

2   Treat callouses, ingrown toenails and do not apply plaster if any skin abrasions have not yet healed.

Application of the plaster itself

1   Apply stockinette, thin cotton wool, allowing stockinette to hang over toes until plaster of Paris is completed.

2   Apply compressed felt, with sides trimmed down, to ankle, heel and front of ankle. A shape may be cut so that a piece of felt covers the sole of the foot and the felt then wraps around from the heel to the front of the ankle. Do not overlap felt as this will act as a pressure area or the padding may shift under the plaster if it is too loose. Apply all materials evenly.

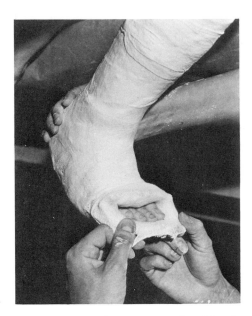

Fig. 8.15

3 Wind wet plaster around ankle first. Do not use a figure eight. The 'holder' keeps the foot at right ankles or more whilst this plaster hardens slightly. It should be applied with firm tension to hold the foot from slipping.
4 Apply a plaster from toes to below the knee holding the foot at right angles or more. TEST that the angle of dorsiflexion used in the plastering can be obtained passively with the child's knee straight.
5 Slabs of plaster are put on along the back of the leg up to the toes. The holder keeps the toes *dorsiflexed* and spread out and presses into the centre of the metatarsal arch. The dorsiflexed toes holds the long arch firmly.
6 Mould the plaster and dent it slightly on either side of the tendon Achilles. The holder must not let the calcaneous slip whilst this is being done. The calcaneus is being kept in the centre, with the T.A. centre.
7 Final plaster around foot ankle and to below the knee (about 1 inch).
8 Smooth and mould plasters to leg. Turn the top plasters back so that you can see all of the child's toes. Cut it at the sides to do this and also cut the stockinette and turn that backwards to reveal toes (Fig. 8.15).
9 Reinforce the sole of the plaster or use a plaster boot for walking. A small flat heel may be set into the plaster. The plaster must cover the toes underneath and hold them in dorsiflexion to avoid toe clenching the edge of the plaster.
10 The plaster must be given about 3 days to set. Check circulation by pressure on toes and observing immediate return of colour. Blue toes indicates the need to have the plaster removed immediately.
11 Valium or other sedative may be needed for the first night in plaster. The strong pull of the child's hypertonic muscles may make him restless.
12 Lift blankets off the child's feet by use of a cradle. Keep the child *off* his feet, with no crawling, kneeling or standing in damp areas for 3 days.

13 Occasionally spasms of flexion appear in his knees or hips. Use knee gaiters and prone position for the first few days.

14 Keep plasters on for 1 week in young children; 2–3 weeks in older children and 4 weeks in older and very stiff children.

Exercises in plaster Emphasise extension movements of the knee and hip, and back (see Figs. 8.1–8.10) e.g. straight leg lift backwards, knee stretching in sitting, side-lying extension. Weight bearing exercises after 3 days. Standing weight shift from leg to leg sideways and forward and back. Shift the pelvis forward over the weight bearing foot, counteracting hip retraction. Sitting stretch up and stand up 'tall'. Stand walk as much as possible, with weight distributed onto both sides equally. Tilt reactions in standing on rocker board or sponge to increase weight bearing through the leg in plaster.

Exercises out of plaster must be continued with the same aims. Below-knee irons with back stops and if necessary T-straps may be worn for a while. A new plaster cut down the side and stiffened with plastic materials may be used for walking. The plaster 'shell' holds the foot and toes in dorsiflexion over the right angle if possible. The Forest Town boot has been made to this design in South Africa (Appendix).

Use a series of plasters for children who do not maintain correction. Have a short period of exercises and weight bearing before the next plaster is applied. The period between plasters has been from 2 years to a few weeks in different cases. Athetoids should only wear a plaster for a week at a time in case of involuntary movements within the plaster.

Foot and knee plasters have been applied simultaneously by Burns, but de Rijke, Hare and others prefer below-knee plasters and knee plasters to be separated. After removal of plasters from hip and knee the child often needs exercises particularly in water, bandaging of knees and treatment of knee swelling as well as long leg caliper.

Cooperation of the parents must be obtained for good results thus:

1 Explain the purpose of the plaster and the importance of their help and encouragement to the child to wear the plaster for short periods.

2 They should check the circulation often be warned about possible restlessness and have a sedative for the child.

3 Parents should protect the plaster and allow drying for 3 days. Child may sit with his leg or legs on cushions protected by waterproof material. An old sock, plaster boot or plastic covering may be used to cover plaster.

4 Parents carry out home exercises and later as much standing and walking as possible.

5 Tell parents when the plaster comes off and they should know when their child is coming home with a plaster before hand or they may think he has broken a leg!

6 If child's toes go blue, or if there is extreme pain and upset, the plaster *must* be removed by soaking it off in a bucket of warm water.

CHAPTER 9

THERAPEUTIC GROUP WORK

The child's need for group activities has long been recognised in the habilitation of handicapped children. Motor handicapped children are often isolated from their peers. They may not be able to run up and join a group of children, put an arm round a friend or even push away an annoying child. Parents find it difficult to bring the handicapped child into contact with other children whether normal or handicapped. Children need group treatment for contact with other children, sharing an activity with others, feeling part of a group and responding to competition and cooperation. Group work in therapy as well as in education offers opportunities for the child's social and emotional development.

Groups have been used in a variety of ways:

In speech therapy for stimulation of communication and development of speech and language.

In occupational therapy for perceptual training, for play involving perceptual motor function, for recreation, social interaction and learning to play a game involving rules and taking turns and so on.

In physiotherapy for training children with a specific diagnosis to carry out a set of exercises, for games involving gross motor activity, for swimming and activities in water, and various sports for the disabled.

As the aims of these different therapy groups overlap it is possible to carry out *interdisciplinary groups* of two kinds:

Playgroups, including toy libraries, adventure playgrounds, special nursery schools, 'opportunity groups' or nurseries, are orientated to each child's developmental levels and special problems. The therapists may advise or themselves work in the group setting, stimulating a few or occasionally all the children with play activities which involve gross motor, fine motor, perceptual and speech and language activities. She may be in the playroom or nursery, relating to one child with specific problems and may or may not also bring in other children in the same activity.

The children may all be in the same room and may or may not feel themselves to belong to the same group in all activities.

Songs, storytime, percussion band, games and music may be the only sessions when all the children carry out the same activity. Therapists are also working with teachers, psychologists, child care staff, nursery nurses, nurses and parents in the therapeutic play groups.

The Structured Group works to treat or train a specific area of function. These groups integrate the gross motor, fine motor, perceptual, speech and language activities, but with more focus on any one of these areas. This focus may be on the major handicap of the children in the group, say motor handicap in cerebral palsied children. The focus may be on a specific area of function in one group session, whereas the focus will be on another area for that same group in other group sessions.

These structured interdisciplinary groups in Britain have been influenced by the ideas of Petö, Hari, and the work of Cotton [61–66], Seglow [116], Brewer [115] and others who introduced these ideas in Britain [118].

These groups may not follow the full system of the Petö approach, which involves very much more than a group session or group sessions. From studies with the staff of the Cheyne Walk Centre for Spastic Children these structured interdisciplinary group sessions for multiply handicapped children were invaluable and often essential for such children [117].

Some of the main observations are:

1 Individual sessions sometimes create too much pressure on the handicapped child and aggravate the normal or abnormal rebelliousness in a child. In the group such children often cooperate because all the other children present were doing what was expected of them.

2 The one-to-one relationship in individual treatment may be too similar to the one-to-one relationship in the mother–child situation. This is normal in children under 3-year developmental level. Physically handicapped children, however, are often over this age and need to relate to their peers *even though* their physical function may still be under a 3-year developmental level.

Although a child may need some 'private tuition' in his school life and some deprived children and severely subnormal children may still need this one-to-one relationship, many more need to 'grow out' of it emotionally and socially. Perhaps some of those who refuse to cooperate may be protesting at the dependency felt on being handled by the therapists all the time in this one-to-one situation.

3 In the group, children follow instructions and imitate the other children. Imitation helps the mentally slower or partially hearing children to understand what is required of them. In addition, the children in groups are observed to instruct and help each other carry out the programme of work.

4 Speech is stimulated as the adult's concentration on all the children seemed to take off the 'pressure' on one child to speak.

5 Concentration of the children who were working at their own pace was great. The attention span was far longer than in individual sessions, children worked hard in groups lasting one and a half hours whilst in individual treatment for only 20–40 minutes.

6 The programme consists of integrating aspects of physiotherapy, occupational therapy, speech therapy together with group work. It is planned by the team but carried out by one therapist and one or two aids or assistants. In this way a number of children are helped at the same time

with economy on staff and on time spent getting children to and from each therapy department, as well as on time required to establish rapport with each different professional.

7 Physiotherapists, occupational therapists, speech therapists, teachers, and nursery nurses welcome interdisciplinary groups as they can then see the total child and the relationship of their speciality to those of the others in his total function. On planning and using the structured group session the different disciplines are made to share their knowledge with one another so that practical integrated group activities can be created. Different disciplines have then to clarify their main aims with each child and make certain they are understood by everyone in the planning of the programme and in its execution. It is not possible for each professional to convey all her expertise to the other different disciplines, but rather to learn how to discover the overlap of her particular discipline with others. In this way the overlap becomes a practical achievement and enriches the teamwork.

GENERAL MANAGEMENT OF GROUPS

Number of children   This varies according to the numbers of children in each centre, school or institution, from whom selections may be made. No matter how many children are in a group, they must be 'involved' and preferably participating.

Staff   One staff member leads the group with another assisting her. The assistant should be from another discipline. If the children are all severely handicapped, more help may be indicated. However, the adults present must be kept to a minimum, or their one-to-child relationship rather than a child-to-child relationship may occur. The leader may alternate with her assistant each week or alternate days in conducting the group.

   All assistants must work under the leader and not divert the child's attention away from the group by private conversation with them or with each other.

Venue   The group is best done in the child's own classroom or where there are no unfamilar distractions and a 'coming and going' of adults or other children.

Arrange children during the group session so that they can see the leader of the group at all times, and also so that the children see each other. Semi-circles or L-shaped seating arrangements are best, but the positions will change in a class with particular motor activities and mobility exercises.

Length of sessions should be planned for 1 to 2 hours depending on the children's ability to continue participating, and the programme of work.

Frequency   Group sessions are best done daily or three times a week depending on aims of the group programme. Some aims only require twice a week. The main object is that the children work together for not less than three times a week so that they know each other and develop a group dynamic.

Behaviour   If a child refuses to join in, make sure that the programme is not too difficult for him. If it is not, let him watch for a while, ignoring him. The other children may be given a particularly pleasant activity or they may occasionally be told 'let's do that again for so-and-so to try as well'. Other ideas may be offered by the parent or team members who know the child. However, if non-participation continues or if the child seems oblivious to other children and group work, the group cannot 'carry' him indefinitely. He may not be ready or not suitable for group treatments, and this is not always obvious in the beginning.

Children with behaviour problems may become disruptive to the group. Hyperkinetic children may be particularly difficult. However, try a trial period of partial sessions with the group, increase to full sessions and the techniques above. Disturbed children may settle down and join in with the others. Finally good selection of children and programme planning makes organised management easier.

SELECTION OF CHILDREN

The basis for selection varies and ideas are still developing. The early days of group treatment both for staff and children seem to be easier if the disparity between the children is not great. A hemiplegic group with children at the walking level and at approximately the same chronological age and intelligence is a simple one to arrange for staff who are inexperienced in group therapy. The hemiplegic group might enlarge itself to encompass other diagnostic types of cerebral palsy who have asymmetry. Mental levels may be varied. A variety of developmental levels among motor developmentally delayed children may be contained in one group.
The following points influencing selection may be helpful.

PROBLEMS OF CHILDREN

Motor problems

Selection of children according to diagnosis is not usually helpful. Select the children according to their problems. Although it is difficult to generalise them, motor problems are usually some or all of the following:

1   Head control—postural fixation, particularly in the upright position.
2   Head and trunk in midline, symmetrical arm and leg postures.
3   Head and trunk counterpoising so that arms and legs can move into various asymmetrical postures or movements.
4   Grasp to hold on, and grasp and release.
5   Corrective movements and postures for any recurring abnormal positions of any joints; e.g., in spastics or athetoids, elbow flexion, shoulder retraction, hip extension or semiflexion, adduction, knee flexion, equinis feet.
6   Form of locomotion.
7   Ability to sit or stand.
8   Ability to rise from the floor or from a chair.

It is possible, say, to have a 'pre-sitting group' with a selection of motor activity building up to sitting, prone to hands and knees and weight bearing on feet with trunk support (see developmental channels on (Fig. 5.1, 0–6 months level). It is possible to have a group on 'sitting and pre-walking' with activities taken from the channels of development of 6–12 months (Fig. 5.1) or an ambulant group, 12 months and over (Fig. 5.1) The motor abilities selected for training will depend on the children with these problems. It is obviously essential to have assessments of the problems. The other aspects of function in the child should be considered although motor problems are primary.

Age of child

Children should be around the same chronological age, as their developmental levels alone will offer a range of children. It is sometimes an unhappy situation if a large boy of 11 with a developmental level of say, sitting equal to about 6–9 months normal level is in a group with 3-year-olds also at this developmental level.

Mental level

The mental level should not cross too wide a spectrum. Some prefer keeping intelligent children in one group whilst others find it useful to 'mix' as the mentally handicapped child will imitate the intelligent child in carrying out the motor activity or other activities which do not demand high intelligence. Mentally deficient children may also be better at movement than say a severely physically handicapped, intelligent athetoid, thus a 'balance' is obtained in the work programme.

Personality and behaviour

Personality of the children is rarely a consideration unless a child is excessively disruptive and management ideas for behaviour fail (see above).

Other handicaps

Deaf, partially sighted or blind children may find it more difficult to join a group if the focus is on the motor handicap. However, again some athetoids with high frequency hearing loss and some spastics with partial hearing have responded well to groups through imitation, lip reading and other visual clues, as well as the fact that a good group session focussed on problems other than specific hearing problems. Severely subnormal children may be too oblivious of the group dynamics being used and remain in their own world, and be unsuitable for such group work.

It must be remembered that factors for selection are still being explored by those working with groups.

Whatever the basis for selection the 'answers' to the best way to select children finally rests on whether group programmes of work can be created by the staff and on the ability of the leader of the group to weld her group of children together, so that they work together and there is a group spirit.

THE PROGRAMME

1   This must be prepared before the group commences.

2   It can be modified once used and *must* be changed as the children change and progress.

3   The group leader must have the programme in front of her so that she does not delay and lose any group 'impetus' and collaboration gained. She must know 'what comes next'.

4   The programme should not be too long, but it is better to spend more time on each item. The items are after all only chosen because they are to be trained and repetition is needed.

5   Occasionally, have an easy item already achieved, as well as items *within* the capacity of the children. If the children experience a successful achievement this motivates them further.

6   Use action songs to carry out motor activities for the children, as they use the same songs each time, their familiarity is often appreciated. For many handicapped children, the programme should contain familiar elements, either songs, the playleader, the room, the time of day or days of week and the general outline. However, the activities must gradually develop and change and not remain so predictable that the children do not progress.

Items of the programme

The details of the programme must be worked out and if necessary written out before the group session begins. The group leader must not be hesitant about the 'next item on the programme' as this disorganises the group concentration and motivation.

The programme and its further modifications must be assessed and re-assessed, not only by the group leader, but also together with the other professional workers in the centre. Ongoing consultations are necessary to make sure that the items selected for the children motivate ALL the children and that any child is not 'carried' as a non-participant for too long.

Select items from the treatment suggestions in the chapters on developmental training and the problems of deformity. Give preference to those items which do not depend on holding or handling the child or there may be too many adults required. Too many adults present disrupts the growing child–child relationships in the group. Select items which are at first easy and become more difficult as the children develop in the group programme. In addition, such selected items may be used in groups to show some children ahead of the others. This motivates the others to work towards these higher levels, which they can observe in their peers. In this way the therapist can have children at different levels of motor development in one group. She must have items selected so that they 'build up' a particular motor ability.

For example:
All the children sit around a large table. Children at 3–6 months developmental level of sitting will have to lean their trunks against the table and grasp a horizontal bar attached to the table or grasp a slatted table. The children from 6–9 months level do not lean against the table, but only grasp the support and the children from 9–12 months who can sit alone, do so with their hands at their sides or on their laps.

Similarly, standing may be modified from standing leaning against the table with grasp support, stand and grasp, and stand alone.

Also prone lying raise head, prone lying raise head and rise onto elbows, and prone lying raise head and rise onto hands can be included simultaneously. With careful planning and assessment of the children many more examples will be found.

All motor activities must be associated with perceptual experience of direction, spatial relationships, colour, body awareness, various matching activities in relating shapes, sizes, textures as well as speech and language, social awareness and of course the fun of children working and playing together (Fig. 9.1).

Music and movement, songs, action songs, fingerplays and any other children's songs and music must be used for group work. However, as with the other activities, these must be modified to relate to the children's levels of development and interest. Imaginative activities such as 'pretend you are a tree in the wind' or 'let's wave our arms like birds' which are used for children's groups should not be used unless the children understand them and are at the 'let's pretend' level of play development. This is about the 3 year level.

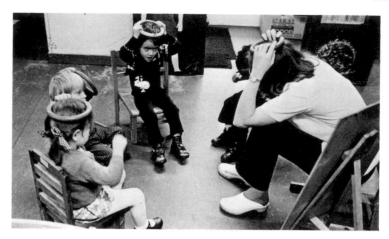

Fig. 9.1

Children's group games and party games may also be adapted and used in group work. Whatever items are selected they MUST NOT be random, but selected according to aims of therapy with each child. There will be aims of therapy which cannot be realised in the group sessions, or not enough in the group sessions. *Individual sessions* will be necessary for the children. However, if the child is well selected and the items well chosen for him in the group, individual sessions may not be essential for him, for a period.

It is not possible to give programmes for groups as these must be composed around the children themselves. However, the following should be included:

1 Start and end with a dressing activity, e.g. taking shoes and socks off, or taking a cardigan off.

2 Fetch and put away any equipment for the group.

3 Use gross motor activities for one session, integrating this with perception and language activities.

4 Use hand classes for a session, integrating this with perception and language activities.

5 Have a meal or tea for the group in order to include feeding training and washing hands.

6 Suggested group games for walkers and non-walkers. These may include crawling hand ball, passing ball or objects in sitting, throwing beanbags into large containers, obstacle course, croquet, ring toss, deck quoits, carpet bowls, shuffle board, rolling balls on the table or floor, ping-pong with the ball attached to a high horizontal wire for ball retrieval and other play activities. Board games should have large counters or handles on the draught pieces or holes for the pieces and other adaptations.

SUMMARY

Interdisciplinary group work is valuable in the treatment of cerebral palsied and motor delayed children. They require consultations between staff:

1   To assess children's functions in all areas before and *during* group sessions.
2   To plan, monitor and progress the items of the group programmes.

It is best for one person to carry out the programme with perhaps other professionals occasionally assisting but *not* interrupting during the group session itself. Adjustments of the programme can be discussed after the session is over.

Teachers and therapists depend on each other to create dynamic group sessions and therefore must work closely together.

DEVELOPMENTAL LEVELS

Function	0–3 months	3–6 months
PRONE		
SUPINE		
SITTING		
STAND		

6–9 *months*   9–12 *months*

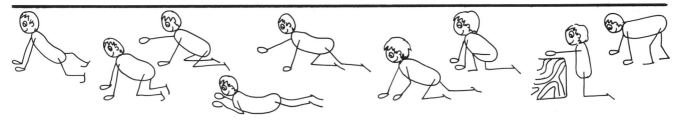

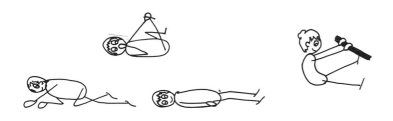

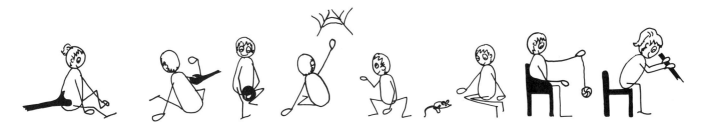

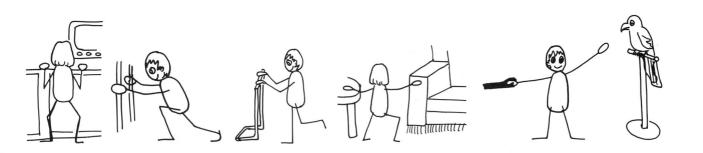

APPENDIX
EQUIPMENT

SELECTION OF EQUIPMENT

Selection and provision of equipment should always be supervised by each child's therapists and medical specialists.

SELECT EQUIPMENT ACCORDING to the following considerations.

1 Assessment of the child's disabilities and abilities especially emerging 'unreliable' abilities. The correct amount of aid makes it possible for him to carry out tasks otherwise impossible, but too much aid prevents his own participation and development of emerging ability.

2 Assessment of the child's deformities or threatening deformities. Good alignment in any apparatus and correction of abnormal postures must be maintained during the use of the equipment. For example standing may be correct in a standing box, but become abnormal on hand function in standing; sitting may be upright in a push-chair with special modifications but become abnormal when the chair is pushed by an adult!

3 Good design of equipment takes account of adjustments for child's growth, removal of supports with increasing ability, a variety of modifications for different children in a clinic/school, be as portable as possible and look as normal as possible. Simple designs easily adjusted by busy parents and staff are desirable.

ONGOING SUPERVISION IS IMPORTANT TO check the following:

1 Measurements of the child as he grows so that equipment is not too small.

2 Value of the equipment in relation to achievements gained in therapy and daily care. Once again equipment must facilitate independence not substitute for it.

3 Unexpected social problems such as equipment being too cumbersome in a home or school; isolating the child from a family group too much; proving too fragile and requiring expense, time and worry on the part of people caring for the child, and other considerations of a similar kind.

Home visits are a great help in discovering these problems as parents may not report these difficulties after 'all the efforts made' by staff to assess, provide and check the equipment in a clinic.

4 Provision of equipment, designs and new ideas change with research and general administrative progress in helping the handicapped and this may help the particular child at the re-assessments.

Equipment lists and related information may be obtained from various

244

voluntary organisations, other parents of handicapped children, Departments of Health, Social Services and Education in local authorities or other Government departments and equipment lists from various Medical Equipment firms, Toy manufacturers and education suppliers.

Consult the following:

Disabled Living Foundations, 346 Kensington High Street, London W14.
Equipment for the Disabled—National Fund for Research into Crippling Diseases.   2 Foredown Drive, Portslade, Sussex, particularly *The Disabled Child*,   Wisbeach A., and *Wheelchairs and Outdoor Transport, Hoists*.
Handling the Cerebral Palsied Child at home, Finnie N., Heinemann Medical, London.
Handicapped Adventure Playground Association, 3 Oakley Gardens, London SW3.
Paediatric Group of Physiotherapists, c/o C.S.P. Bedford Row, London WC1.
Paediatric Group of Occupational Therapists, British O.T. Association, 20 Rede Place, London W2.
Voluntary societies concerned with the care of the disabled child especially:
  The Spastics Society, Information and Supplies Officer, 12 Park Cresent, London W1. Assessment Unit, 16 Fitzroy Square, London W1.
  Toy Library Association, Sunley House, Gunthorpe Street, London E16.
  National Society for Mentally Handicapped Children, Pembridge Hall, 17 Pembridge Square, London W2.
  Muscular Dystrophy Group of Great Britain, (Handbook) 35 Macaulay Road, Clapham, London, SW4.
  Downs Babies Centre, 40 Lodge Hill Road, Birmingham.

BASIC EQUIPMENT

Imaginitive parents and therapists require a mat, chairs of different sizes, tables of different sizes and everyday objects in the home especially in the kitchen, and also use of grass, sand, water, leaves and so on outside the house.

Additional equipment is selected *according to the children* and this is usually

Wedges other sponge rubber shapes or firm cushions.

Sponge rubber rolls of different diameters or cardboard cylinders padded with sponge-blankets. Cover wedges, shapes, rolls with waterproof and washable material. Canvas wedges are also available (Fig. 1a, b). Diameters of rolls are from 10″ for prone lying, chest support, to take weight on elbows or hands; take weight on knees, or sit astride roll in squatting position or for sitting a small child. Large diameters for tilt reactions, arm saving reactions; lower to standing; standing arm support

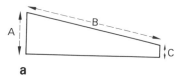

a

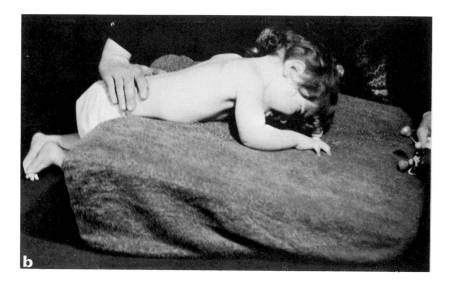

Fig 1a Measurements for wedge for
prone lying, arms over edge 'A'.
A, Measurement from axilla to wrist.
B, Measurement from axilla to 2 in
above ankle. C, Length of top of foot.
b, Use wedge for weightbearing on
knees or reversed for weightbearing
on elbows or on hands, stimulation of
head raise, and use of hands on the
floor. Straps may be needed to hold
the child on the wedge.

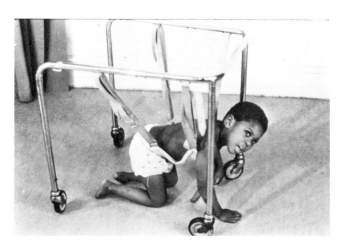

Fig. 2 A crawler.

on roll (p. 162). Sizes $30'' \times 10''$; $30'' \times 15''$; $30'' \times 20''$; $45'' \times 20''$ (Price Bros & Co., Wellington, Somerset).

Large inflatable balls including beach balls may be used instead of rolls. Diameters $44''$; $32''$. Small beachballs of various sizes are usually obtained by therapists.

Chairs and tables   See Chapter 6 on the Development of Sitting which includes beanbag chairs; inflatable chairs; foam shaped seats; floor seats; baby relax and other baby chairs; canvas seats; roll converted into a seat and saddle seat; engine and desk; adjustable corner seat with tray fitment and simple chairs with non-slip seats backs and sides (removable) of different sizes to fit different children. The Peto idea of a slatted chair is also useful for training various motor tasks well as sitting (p. 126) Toilet seats, potties, lavatory seats. Car seats. Bath seats. Portable shower seat on wheels are available on the market. Variable height tables should be obtained whenever possible. Cut out tables should also be adjustable.

Crawlers   A canvas sling under the child's abdomen and supports on casters is essentially the basic principle used in crawlers. Many adjustments may be required, e.g. straps to hold the thighs in flexion and prevent 'shooting' into abnormal extension; straps to stop thighs or arms pushing into the area beneath the child's abdomen; small wedge, straps or cushion to stop child sliding off crawler and adjustments of the height of the body support so that the length of the child's arms reaches the distance to the floor from that abdominal–chest support. Platforms on wheels, wedges on wheels (castors) or toy creations such as the dolphin on casters are also used by some children for crawling on hands only, on knees only, or on hands-and-knees.

Apparatus for supported standing   Various standing frames are available (Fig. 3). The child can stand and hold parallel or vertical bars; backs of chairs or walking aids are also used.

NOTE   Standing aids do not train standing unless the aid is vertical with the line of gravity going from the child's head (ear) down to just behind his ankle. Adjust the foot pieces of the skis or straps of the stabiliser (Standing Frame to thigh or to knee) to obtain the correct alignment. Any aid with a forward or a backward lean is only of value to correct flexed hips by strapping, knees by knee pieces and feet held at right angles by a board and/or foot pieces.

Prone Boards/Forward Standing Frame attached at a forward angle to a table for schoolwork or hand activities corrects abnormal postures of the legs, keeps the trunk straight and stimulates head control and arm function. Standing boards or beds do the same but are used more for ball throwing, arm exercises and periods of passive stretching of flexors and plantar flexors. Large pommels or other ideas may be incorporated to keep legs apart and also occasionally externally rotated. None of these aids train standing but only give correct postures and prevent deformity (see p. 150).

Walking aids   There are a great variety and they should be carefully selected.

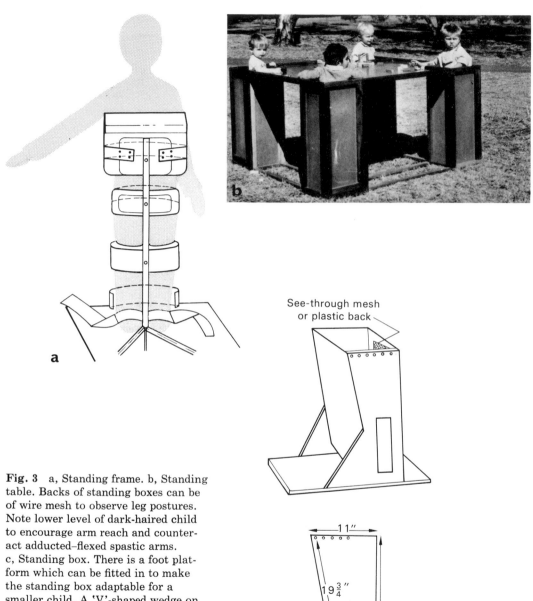

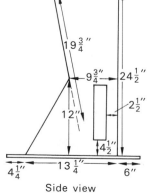

See-through mesh or plastic back

Fig. 3 a, Standing frame. b, Standing table. Backs of standing boxes can be of wire mesh to observe leg postures. Note lower level of dark-haired child to encourage arm reach and counter-act adducted–flexed spastic arms.
c, Standing box. There is a foot plat-form which can be fitted in to make the standing box adaptable for a smaller child. A 'V'-shaped wedge on the platform keeps the child's feet in a good position. A ledge is attached to both sides of the box and the bars of the tray are made to slide over this. The tray is slid on and fixed in position with bolts fitting into holes on the side of the box. These holes and wire mesh at the back enable the therapist to see the child is in a good position. The rim of the tray is about $\frac{3}{4}''$ high.

Side view

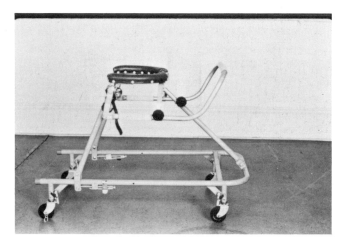

Fig. 4.

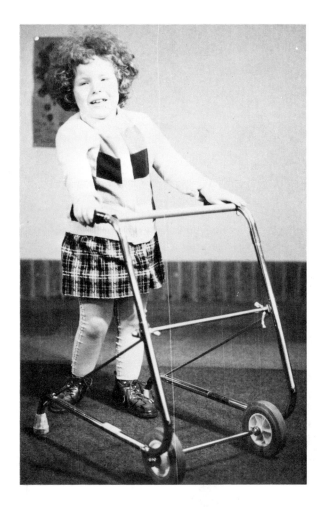

Fig. 5

—*With trunk support* given by a padded support to chest or by chest slings attached to overhead. The Amesbury Walker is shown with an adjustable chest to waist support as the child improves his control (Fig. 4).

—*Without trunk support*. A four point walker which can be pushed with grasp on the sides of the child or grasp in front of the child. The Rollator is one example but similar designs exist (Fig. 5).

Toy walkers or doll's prams are very popular. Large soft toys on wheels, large trucks, large toy boxes on castors and similar normal toys should be stable, weighted and checked for size according to the child.

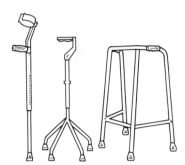

Fig. 6 Walking aids.

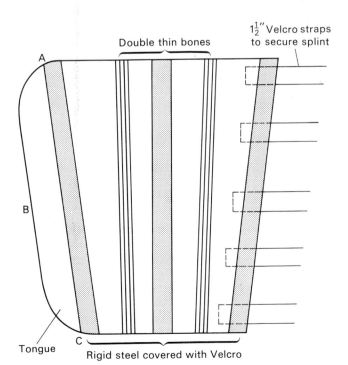

Double thin bones

$1\frac{1}{2}''$ Velcro straps to secure splint

A

B

Tongue

C

Rigid steel covered with Velcro

Fig. 7 Leg gaiter made of white coutil. It is wrapped around the leg bringing velcro straps over the front side of 'B'.

Pushing stable children's or adult's chairs which slide easily but not too quickly as well as boxes on skis and other simple aids also train walking. NOTE Check that wheels on walkers are correct for the child. If they 'run away' preventing correct postures and establishment of the child's own control of his balance, use the walkers with crutch tips at each of the four points, ski sliders or other modifications. Various walkers without wheels are on the market *Crutches, elbow crutches, quadripods, tripods* and *thick based sticks* are used for selected children (Fig. 6). Frequently progress is made from crutches to sticks. Check length, hand grasps and stability. Some sticks (of wood) may be linked together with a centre piece for initial stability.

NOTE All walking aids should be checked for height so that the child does not grasp them with abnormal shoulder hunching, excessive flexion of the elbows and radial deviation of wrists. If grasp is not possible without these abnormalities try a walking aid which requires pushing with flat hands and straight elbows, or use a chair.

Parallel bars These should be adjustable in height, sometimes in width. Hand slides are used if the child cannot grasp and release to use the parallel bars. A chair at the end of the bars may be used for training standing up from sitting. Eversion boards, foot prints and abduction boards have been placed between the bars when needed. Do not use parallel bars for spastics who grasp in excessive flexion which cannot be eliminated by lowering the bars for elbow extension.

Appliances for correct posture in standing; weightbearing; trunk control, and to 'weight' the feet of unstable athetoids or ataxics with below-knee appliances:

Long leg calipers (braces) which have thigh bands, knee pieces and fit into boots. These keep knees straight. Knees may unlock to allow sitting.

There may be pelvic bands and adjustments to lock/unlock hip to keep hips straight and facing forward, with some abduction. Abduction-external rotation is not often possible in spastics. A rotator coil may help, but could twist the knee too much. Also, T-straps and back or front locks attached to the long leg brace at the ankle (see below-knee iron).

Below-knee irons. with attachment to the heel of the child's boot, under the heel or having a joint opposite the ankle. The iron locks against a stop to prevent plantarflexion (back stop) or to prevent dorsiflexion (front stop). T-strap inside to counter pronation. T-strap outside to counter varus.

Knee gaiters or polythene knee moulds, plaster knee moulds to keep knees straight (Fig. 7).

Abduction pants to keep legs apart. It may need stiffening with some light plastic material if adduction is strong (Fig. 8) [94].

Elbow gaiters which keep elbows straight for correct arm push and grasp of walkers and other poles in other functions (Fig. 9).

Boots may have to be
1 Padded at the tongue to fit well around the ankle.

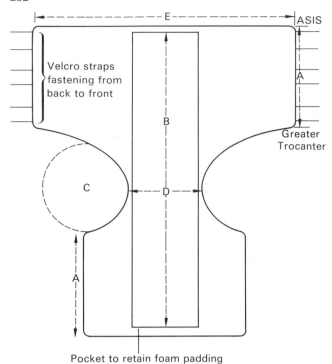

Fig. 8 Inside view of abduction pants, made of white coutil and lined with waterproofing, including the pocket. Fit very firmly around the pelvis.

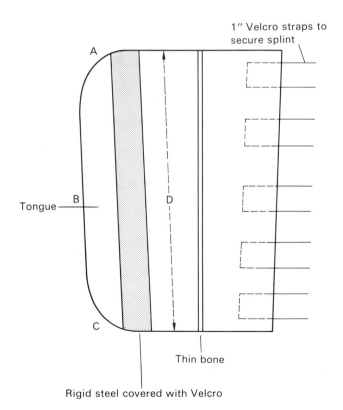

Fig. 9 Arm splint made of white coutil. Wrap splint around arm bringing velcro straps over side 'B'.

2   Have a strap to cross the front of the ankle to press heel well down.

3   Have an inside mould at the inside arch to control valgus.

4   Have an external heel extension on the inner side of the sole to prevent pronation (valgus) of the foot: on the outer side of sole to prevent supination (varus)

5   Have a raise on the heel, with a flare on the inner side for valgus; outer side for varus.

6   Special boots may be made in the design of 'The Forest Town Boot' (Fig. 10).

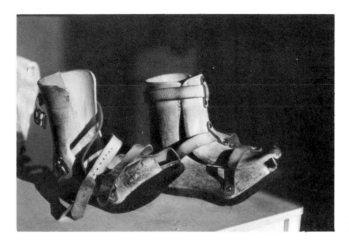

Fig. 10   Forest Town Boot.

7   Boot may have a sole raised to provoke forward weight shift to step, or to stretch heel cords. Sometimes just removal of the heels and thick soles stops toe walking in a mild spastic child.

8   Boots or shoes may have a weighted base to add stability for, say, ataxics.

9   Stiffening on the boot leather may be given on the inside or outside to stop the foot rolling over into either pronation or supination respectively.

10   Toes of boots often have to be protected with thick rubbers, plastic coatings or metal to avoid the frequent wearing of the leather in 'toe walkers' or 'crawlers' who are just beginning to walk.

11   Crawling children or non-walkers have boots and shoes to keep their feet warm, without any modifications. Booties or 'running shoes' stay on their feet better.

NOTE   Putting on and off shoes and boots is facilitated by the use of laces down to the toes as in Shoo-shoos and Piedro shoes. Toes can then be held flat during application of boots. Velcro instead of laces make it possible for some children to put their own shoes on and off. A tab on the back of the boot helps the child to pull on his boot.

Stairs with bannisters can be part of the physiotherapy department. Stairs should vary in height.

Ramps, uneven ground, various floor surfaces should be available for training walking.

Mirrors to floor level may be a help in training sitting, standing and walking.

Aids to activities of daily living Consult occupational therapists.

Feeding

Dycem mat, long-handled spoons, spoons of different sizes, metal and unbreakable plastic spoons, rubberzote and other handles, dishes with and without sides. 'Keep-dishes-warm'. Suction rubbers to hold bowl on table. Bibs. Cups; Non-slip, weighted, sponge rubber suctions to hold cup and straw steady, baby mugs with non-spill aids and training lids with small opening. Mugs with two handles and one handle which is easy to grasp.

Dressing

Velcro. Zips and special designs. Detachable fronts for children who drool or mess. Large buttons, hooks or other fastenings.

Bathing

Non-slip mat in bath, small bath within large bath. Inflatable chair propped in bath, (Suzy) neck supports, bath seats hooked on sides. Liquid bath cleansers to avoid soaping when there are difficulties.

Toilet See chairs and sitting, pp. 127–128.

Sleeping bags, cots, baby toys etc. as for normal babies.

Prams, pushchairs and baby buggies. As for normal children but check postures more carefully.

Wheelchairs A variety are available. References should be made to those given in the beginning of this Appendix.

The principles of correct sitting discussed in Chapter 6 on Development of Sitting and chairs should be applied to the child in wheelchairs with the added considerations of:

a   Can he propel the chair himself or must it be pushed? Can he transfer?

b   Facilities of the child's home for containing a wheelchair—stairs, doorways, sizes of rooms, use of table heights available, etc.

c   Is the wheelchair useful indoors, outdoors or both?

d   Can the wheelchair 'grow' with the child. What modifications?

e   Can the wheelchair be transported, stored, put on public transport?

(Reference should be made to the wheelchair research programme under Dr. Stephen Jarvis which is in preparation at the Wolfson Centre, Mecklenburgh Square, London WC1)

Special aids in the Classroom See References beginning of Appendix Typewriters; 'possum' and other electronic aids to communication; page turners; communication boards; pencil holders, page and book holders, clips for drawing pages etc.

Aids to mobility other than walkers, crawlers and wheelchairs.

Chailey chariots; tricycles with adaptations. Hand-propelled tricycles. Prone tricycles. Corner seat on casters. A variety of mobility toys is in development by engineers, research workers, parents, therapists and toy manufacturers.

See Adventure Playgrounds, brochure reference above.

Lady Hoare Trust for Physically Disabled Children, 2 Milford House, 7 Queen Anne Street, London W1; Disabled Living Foundation; Equipment for the Disabled.

General

Helmets to protect the child's head if he falls frequently. Toy catalogues. Toy libraries catalogues for appropriate toys. Gym apparatus (balls, hoops, ropes, climbing apparatus). Adventure playground apparatus, playthings and equipment. Rocking boards, rocking toys, swings, slides, climbing frames

Thumb splint (Fig. 11).

NOTE Treatment tables in physiotherapy should be high for some physio-therapy techniques and low for training the child to get off the treatment table into standing, to climb etc.

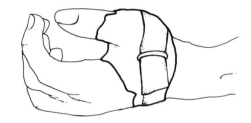

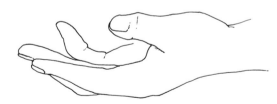

Fig. 11 Thumb splint to correct adducted–flexed thumb. A cock-up wrist splint to midline may be incorporated if palm flexion is excessive. Figure of eight thumb splint at base of thumb and over the wrist in soft pigskin or simply a handkerchief may be adequate for babies and young children.

REFERENCES

CHAPTER 1. AETIOLOGY, DIAGNOSIS, NORMAL AND ABNORMAL DEVELOPMENT, NEUROPHYSIOLOGY

1 GORDON N. (1976) *Paediatric Neurology for the Clinician.* Heinemann Medical Books, London.
2 WOODS G. (1975) *The Handicapped Child.* Blackwell Scientific Publications, Oxford.
3 ASHER & SCHONELL (1950) A survey of 400 cases of cerebral palsy in childhood. *Arch. Dis. Child.* **25,** 360.
4 INGRAM T.T.S. (1964) *Paediatric Aspects of Cerebral Palsy.* Livingstone, Edinburgh.
5 FOLEY J. (1969) *Cerebral Palsy and the Young Child.* Ed. Blencowe. E. & S. Livingstone, Edinburgh.
6 BAX M.C.O. (1964) Terminology and classification of cerebral palsy. *Dev. Med. & Child Neurol.* **6,** 295.
7 HENDERSON J. (1964) *Cerebral Palsy in Childhood and Adolescence.* E. & S. Livingstone, Edinburgh and London.
8 DENHOFF E. (1967) *Cerebral Palsy—The Preschool Years.* C. C. Thomas, Springfield, Ill.
9 CROTHERS B. & PAINE R.S. (1959) *The Natural History of Cerebral Palsy.* Harvard University Press, Cambridge, Mass.
10 COLLIS E., COLLIS R., DUNHAM, HILLIARD & LAWSON (1956) *The Infantile Cerebral Palsies.* Heinemann, London.
11 PERLSTEIN M.A. (1950) Medical aspects of cerebral palsy. Incidence, etiology, pathogenesis. *Am. J. Occup. Therapy,* **4,** 76.
12 PHELPS W.M. (1949) *Description and differentiation of types of cerebral palsy. Nerv. Child,* **8,** 107.
13 ANDRE-THOMAS, ST ANNE DARGASSIES, CHESNI Y. (1960) *Neurological examination of the infant.* Heinemann—Spastic Society, London.
14 BOBATH B. & BOBATH K. (1975) *Motor Development in the Different Types of Cerebral Palsy.* Heinemann, London.
15 BOBATH K. (1971) The normal postural reflex mechanism and its deviation in children with cerebral palsy. *Physiotherapy,* Nov.
16 BOBATH K. (1966) *The Motor Deficit in Patients with Cerebral Palsy.* Heinemann, London.
17 BOBATH BERTA (1965) *Abnormal Postural Reflex Activity caused by Brain Lesions.* Heinemann, London.
18 FIORENTINO M. (1972) *Normal and Abnormal Development.* C. C. Thomas, Springfield, Ill.
19 FIORENTINO M. (1963) *Reflex Testing Methods for Evaluation of C.N.S. Development.* C. C. Thomas, Springfield, Ill.
20 GESELL A. (1966) *The First Five Years of Life.* 5th edn. Methuen, London.

21 GESELL A. & ARMATRUDA (1954) *Developmental Diagnosis.* Hoeber, Harper, New York.

22 SHERIDAN M.D. (1975) *The Developmental Progress of Infants and Young Children*, 3rd edn. HMSO, London.

23 SHERIDAN M.D. (1973) *Children's Developmental Progress. Birth—5 years.* NFER Publishing Company, Windsor.

24 GRIFFITHS R. (1954) *The Abilities of Babies.* University of London Press, London.

25 HOLT K. (1975) (ed.) *Movement and Child Development.* (Ed) Chapters by Holt; Rosenbloom; Wyke; Brand and Rosenbaum; Rosenbaum, Barnitt and Brand; Rosenbloom and Horton. Heinemann—Spastics International Medical Publications, London.

26 ILLINGWORTH R.S. (1975) *Basic Developmental Screening 0–2 years.* Blackwell Scientific Publications, Oxford.

27 ILLINGWORTH R.S. (1972) *The Development of the Infant and Young Child. Normal and Abnormal.* 5th edn. Livingstone, Edinburgh and London.

28 ILLINGWORTH R.S. (1953) *The Normal Child.* Churchill, London.

29 MARTIN J.P. (1967) *The Basal Ganglia and Posture.* Pitman Medical Publications, London.

30 MARTIN J.P. (1965) Tilting reactions and disorders of the basal ganglia. *Brain*, **88,** 855.

31 MILANI-COMPARETTI A. & GIDONI E.A. (1967) Routine developmental examination in normal and retarded Children. *Dev. Med. & Child Neurol*, **9,** 625.

32 PAINE R.S. & OPPE T.E. (1966) *Neurological Examination of Children.* Heinemann Books—Spastic International Publications, London.

33 PAINE R.S. (1964) The evolution of infantile postural reflexes in the presence of chronic brain syndromes. *Dev. Med. & Child Neurol.* **6,** 345.

34 PEIPER A. (1963) *Cerebral Function in Infancy and Childhood.* Consultants Bureau, New York. Also Pitman Medical, London.

35 MCGRAW M. (1943) *The Neuromuscular Maturation of the Human Infant.* Columbia University Press.

36 TWITCHELL T.E. (1965) Variation and abnormalities of motor development. *Phys. Ther. Rev.* **45** (5) 424.

37 TWITCHELL T.E. (1963) The neurological examination in infantile cerebral palsy. *Dev. Med. Child Neurol.*, **5,** 271.

38 TWITCHELL T.E. (1961) The nature of the motor deficit in double athetosis. *Arch. Phys. Med.* **42,** 63.

39 TOUWEN B.C.L. (1975) *Neurological Development in Infancy.* Drukkerij Grasmeijer & Wijngaard, Groningen, The Netherlands.

40 PRECHTL H.F.R. & BEINTEMA J. (1964) The neurological examination of the full term newborn infant. *Clin. Dev. Med.* No. 12. Heinemann—Spastics Society, London.

41 EGAN D., ILLINGWORTH R.S. & MACKEITH R.C. (1974) *Developmental Screening 0–5 years.* Heinemann—Spastics International Medical Publications, London.

42 VAN BLANKENSTEIN M., WELBERGEN U.R., DE HAAS J.H. (1975) *Development of the Infant.* Heinemann, London.

43 PEARSON P.H. & WILLIAMS C.E. (1972) *Physical Therapy Services in the Developmental Diasabilities.* C. C. Thomas, Springfield, Ill.

44 ROBERTS D.M. (1967) *Neurophysiology of Postural Mechanisms.* Butterworth, London.

45 RUSHWORTH (1961) Posture and righting reflexes. *Cerebral Palsy Bulletin*, **3,** 535.

46 WALSHE F.M.R. (1923) On certain tonic or postural reflexes in hemiplegia. *Brain*, **46,** 2.

47 NORMAL DEVELOPMENT OF MOVEMENT—Issue of *Physiotherapy*, April 1971, London.

CHAPTERS 2–9. TREATMENT PLANNING, THERAPY APPROACHES, ASSESSMENT AND TECHNIQUES

1 COLLES E. (1947) *A Way of Life for the Handicapped Child.* Faber & Faber, London.

2 COLLES E. (1953) Management of cerebral palsy in children. *Medical Illustration,* **7.**

3 SHERIDAN M.D. (1973) *The Handicapped Child and his Home.* National Children's Home, Highbury Park, London.

4 COLLINS J. & BRINKWORTH R. (1973) *Improving Babies with Down's Syndrome,* 5th edn. N.I. Region, National Society for Mentally Handicapped Children. Annadale Ave., Belfast.

5 BLENCOWE S. (1969) (ed.) *Cerebral Palsy and the Young Child.* E. & S. Livingstone, London.

6 DENHOFF E. & ROBINAULT I.P. (1960) *Cerebral Palsy and Related Disorders.* McGraw-Hill, New York.

7 LEVITT S. (1970) Principles of treatment in cerebral palsy. *Fysioterapeuten,* **10.**

8 LEVITT S. & MILLER C. (1973) The interrelationships of speech therapy and physiotherapy in children with neurodevelopmental disorders. *Dev. Med. Child Neurol.,* **15** (2).

9 ELLIS E. (1967) *The Physical Management of Developmental Disorders.* Heinemann—Spastics International Medical Publications, London.

10 SEMANS S. (1966) Principles of treatment in cerebral palsy. *Phys. Ther.,* **46,** 715.

11 FINNIE N. (1974) *Handling the Young Cerebral Palsied Child at Home.* Heinemann, London.

12 PHYSIOTHERAPY ISSUE (1971, September) *Treating the Multiply Handicapped Child.* Chartered Society of Physiotherapy, London.

13 BOBATH B. (1971) Motor development, its effect on general development and application to the treatment of cerebral palsy. *Physiotherapy* **57,** 526.

14 BOBATH K. (1971) The normal postural reflex mechanism and its deviation in children with cerebral palsy. *Physiotherapy* **57,** 515.

15 BOBATH B. (1963) Treatment principles and planning in cerebral palsy. *Physiotherapy,* **49,** 122.

16 SEMANS S. (1967) Bobath approach In *Exploratory and Analytical Survey of Therapeutic Exercise. Am. J. Phys. Med.* **26.** Williams and Wilkins, Baltimore.

17 BOBATH B. & BOBATH K. (1975) Motor development in the different types of cerebral palsy. Heinemann, London.

18 SHEPHERD R. (1974) *Physiotherapy in Paediatrics.* (Cerebral palsy sections are from Bobath.) Heinemann, London.

19 HOLT K.S. (1966) Facts and fallacies about neuromuscular function in cerebral palsy as revealed by electromyography. *Dev. Med. Child Neurol.,* **8,** 255.

20 HOLT K.S. (1965) *Assessment of Cerebral Palsy.* Lloyd-Luke, London.

21 HOLT K.S. & REYNELL J.K. (1967) *Assessment of Cerebral Palsy.* 11. Lloyd-Luke, London.

22 BOWLEY A.H. & GARDINER L. (1969) *The Young Handicapped Child.* E. & S. Livingstone, London.

23 ROBSON P. (1970) Shuffling, hitching, scooting or sliding: some observations in 30 otherwise normal children. *Dev. Med. Child. Neurol.,* **12,** 608.

24 ZUCK F.M., SCHWARTZ P. & JOHNSON M.K. (1952) *Need and resources for stimulating volition of children with cerebral palsy,* and *The progress of cerebral palsy patients under inpatient circumstances,* in *American Academy of Orthopaedic Surgeons Instructional Course Lectures.* Vol. 9. 1952.

25 LEVITT SOPHIE (1976) Stimulation of movement: A review of therapeutic techniques in *Early Management of Handicapping Disorders,* ed. Woodford & Oppe. IRMMH. Rev. of Research and Practice, reprinted from *Movement and*

Child Development, ed. Holt K. Heinemann—Spastics International Medical Publications, London.

26 PHELPS W.M. (1952) The rôle of physical therapy in cerebral palsy and bracing in the cerebral palsies, in *Orthopaedic Appliances Atlas 1*, p. 251, p. 522. Edwards, Ann Arbor.

27 PHELPS W.M. (1953) Personal communication. Childrens Rehab. Inst., Baltimore. U.S.A.

28 EGEL P.F. (1948) *Technique of Treatment for the Cerebral Palsy Child.* C. V. Mosby, St Louis, USA.

29 JACOBSON E. (1938) *Progressive Relaxation.* University of Chicago Press.

30 MARTIN PURDON J. (1967) *The Basal Ganglia and Posture.* Pitman Medical, London.

31 DEAVER G.G. (1956) Cerebral palsy—Methods of treating the neuromuscular disabilities. *Arch. phys. Med.*, **37,** 363.

32 POHL J.F.M. (1950) *Cerebral Palsy.* Bruce, Minneapolis.

33 PLUM P. (1966) Personal communication on his visit to London from Rijkshospital Copenhagen, Denmark. His films of treatment at Cheyne Walk. Spastic Centre.

34 PLUM P. & MOLHAVE A. (1956) Clinical analysis of static and dynamic patterns in cerebral palsy with a view to active correction. *Arch. Phys. Med.*, **37,** 8.

35 ROOD M.S. (1956) Neurophysiological mechanisms utilized in the treatment of neuromuscular dysfunction. *Am. J. Occup. Therapy*, **10** (4) part 2, 220.

36 TARDIEU G. (1973) *The Equinus in Cerebral Palsy.* English edn. C.D.I. Cahiers No. 1, 5. Paris.

37 TARDIEU G. (1973) *Factorial Analysis as an Approach to Cerebral Palsy*, English edn. Cahiers du C.D.I. No. 2 Half year, 7. Paris.

38 FAY T. (1954) Rehabilitation of patients with spastic paralysis. *J. Intern. Coll. Surgeons*, **22,** 200.

39 FAY T. (1954) *Use of Patterns and Reflexes in the Treatment of the Spastic.* Address at Conference, British Council for Welfare of Spastics, London, Sept. 1954.

40 FAY T. (1954) Use of pathological and unlocking reflexes in the rehabilitation of spastics. *Am. J. Phys. Med.*, **33** (6), 347.

41 DOMAN G., DOMAN R. *et al.* (1960) Children with severe brain injuries. Neurological organisation in terms of mobility. *J.A.M.A.*, **174,** 257.

42 BRUNNSTROM S. (1962) Training the adult hemiplegic patient: orientation of techniques to patient's motor behaviour. In *Approaches to Treatment of Patients with Neuromuscular Dysfunction.* 3rd Internat. Congress World Fed. of Occupational Therapists.

43 BRUNNSTROM S. (1956) Methods used to elicit, reinforce and co-ordinate muscular response—Upper motor neurone lesions. APTA–OVR Institute Papers, p. 100. American Physical Therapy Association, New York.

44 KNOTT M. & VOSS D.E. (1968) *Proprioceptive Neuromuscular Facilitation. Patterns and Techniques.* 2nd edn. Harper and Row, Hoeber Medical Division, New York.

45 VOSS D.E. (1972) Proprioceptive Neuromuscular Facilitation. Chapter 5 in *Physical Therapy Services in the Developmental Disabilities*, ed. Pearson & Williams. C. C. Thomas, Springfield, Ill.

46 KABAT H. (1961) Proprioceptive facilitation in therapeutic exercise, in *Therapeutic Exercise*, ed. Licht S. 2nd edn., chapter 13. Licht, New Haven, Connecticut.

47 KABAT H., McLEOD M. & HOLT C. (1959) The practical application of Proprioceptive Neuromuscular Facilitation. *Physiotherapy*, April 1959.

48 COLLIS E. (1953) Course at Queen Mary's Hospital, Carshalton: Personal communication.

49 BOBATH K. & BOBATH B. (1972) Cerebral Palsy, Part 1, and The Neurodevelopmental Approach to Treatment, Part 2, in *Physical Therapy Services in the Developmental Disabilities*, ed. Pearson & Williams. C. C. Thomas, Springfield, Ill.

50 BOBATH B. & BOBATH K. (1964) The facilitation of normal postural reactions and movements in the treatment of cerebral palsy. *Physiotherapy*, **50** (8), 246.

51 BOBATH B. (1967) The very early treatment of cerebral palsy. *Dev. Med. Child Neurol.*, **9** (4), 373.

52 BOBATH B. (1976, 1974) Personal communication. Videotapes.

53 ROOD MARGARET (1962) Use of sensory receptors to activate, facilitate and inhibit motor response, automatic and somatic, in developmental sequence, in *Approaches to the Treatment of Patients with Neuromuscular Dysfunction*, ed. Sattely C. *3rd Int. Congress of World Fed. of Occupational Therapists.*

54 ROOD M. (1974) Notes from Course attended by therapists from Kitchener, Canada. Videotapes at Hamilton, Canada. Notes of students on Course in London and in South Africa.

55 STOCKMEYER S.A. (1972) A sensorimotor approach to treatment. Chapter 4 in *Physical Therapy Services in the Developmental Disabilities*, ed. Pearson & Williams. C. C. Thomas, Springfield, Ill.

56 GOFF B. (1969) Appropriate afferent stimulation. *Physiotherapy*, Vol. LV, 9.

57 STOCKMEYER S.A. (1967) The Rood approach. *Am. J. Phys. Med.*, **46**, No. 1, 900.

58 VOJTA V. (1974) Die Cerebralen Bewegangsstorungen im Sauglingsalter Ferdinand Enke Verlag, Stuttgart.

59 VOJTA V. Lectures and demonstrations on Course in Stockholm; Demonstrations/discussion by Vojta's therapists in Rome, Belgium, Sweden and London, particularly Maresova, Hendrickx and van Mechelin, Jones Barry and Gunn Ursula (1970–1976).

60 HARI M. (1975, 1972, 1968, 1969) Lectures and films at Congresses in Dublin, Oxford, Int. Cerebral Palsy Society and the October 1968 Course at Castle Priory, and Proc. Int. Symposium on the Disabled Child, Brugges, Belgium.

61 COTTON E. (1975) Conductive education and cerebral palsy. The Spastics Society, London.

62 COTTON E. (1974) Improvement in Motor Function with the use of Conductive Education, *Dev. Med. Child Neurol.*, **16,** 637.

63 COTTON E. (1970) Integration of treatment and education in cerebral palsy. *Physiotherapy*, **56** (4), 143.

64 COTTON E. (1968) Conductive education with special reference to severe Athetoids in a non-residential centre. *J. Ment. Subnorm.*, **14** (26), 50.

65 COTTON E. (1965) The Institute for Movement Therapy and School for Conductors, Budapest, Hungary. *Dev. Med. & Child Neurol.*, **17,** 437.

66 COTTON E. (1975) *The Basic Motor Pattern*. The Spastics Society and Three-Day Course at Castle Priory.

67 GILLETTE H.E. (1969) *Systems of Therapy in Cerebral Palsy.* C. C. Thomas, Springfield, Ill.

68 WOLF J.M. (1969) *The Results of Treatment in Cerebral Palsy.* C. C. Thomas, Springfield, Ill.

69 DECKER R. (1962) *Motor Integration.* C. C. Thomas, Springfield, Ill.

70 SNELL E.E. (1955) *Physical Therapy in Cerebral Palsy* (quoting also *Perlstein*) in *Cerebral Palsy*. Eds Cruickshank W. M. and Raus. Syracuse Univ. Press.

71 LEVITT S. (1962) *Physiotherapy in Cerebral Palsy.* C. C. Thomas, Springfield, Ill.

72 LEVITT S. (1969a) Relaxation in Cerebral Palsy (selection of methods from various systems). Paper published in *Proceedings of the International Symposium on the Disabled Child in Brugges, Belgium, Sept.* 1969.

73 LEVITT S. (1969b) *Physiotherapy in Cerebral Palsy and the Young Child*, Chapter 7, ed. Blencowe. E. & S. Livingstone, London.

74 LEVITT S. (1972) *The eclectic approach in cerebral palsy.* Paper given at the Conference of the International Cerebral Palsy Society. April 1972, Oxford.

75 Levitt S. (1974) Common factors in the different systems of treatment in cerebral palsy at Conference of C.D.I. and published in French. C.D.I. Cahier no. 59, Avril-Juin, 1974. Paris.

76 LEVITT S. (1969 to 1975) Lectures on Courses at Cheyne Walk Spastic Centre, London.

77 See Developmental intervention programmes, Motor stimulation in playgroups, opportunity groups, programmes for disadvantaged, mentally retarded or 'slow' children. 'Mother treatments' (Gillette, reference 67).

78 PAINE R.S. (1964) See Charts illustrating 'the evolution of infantile postural reflexes in the presence of chronic brain syndromes', *Dev. Med. Child Neurol.* **6,** 345, and *Neurology* (Minneapolis), **14,** 1036.

79 NATHAN P. (1969) Annotation: Treatment of Spasticity with Peri-neural Injections of Phenol. *Dev. Med. & Child Neurol.* **11,** 384.

80 PEDERSON E. (1969) Spasticity, mechanism, measurement, management. C. C. Thomas, Springfield, Ill.

81 FOLEY J. (1975) Personal communication. Lectures at Cheyne Walk Spastic Centre.

82 HAGBARTH K.-E. & EKLUND G. (1969) The muscle vibrator—a useful tool in neurological therapeutic work. p. 27, *Scan. J. Rehab. Med.*, **1,** 26.

83 SAMILSON R.L. (1975) (ed.) *Orthopaedic Aspects of Cerebral Palsy*, Heinemann—Spastics International Publications, London.

84 SHARRARD W.J.W. (1971) *Paediatric Orthopaedics and Fractures.* Blackwell Scientific Publications, Oxford.

85 DE RIJKE H. (1967–1973) Lectures at Cheyne Walk Spastic Centre, London.

86 HELD R. (1965) Plasticity in sensory motor systems. *Scientific American*, **213** (5), 84.

87 LEVITT S. (1970) Adaptation of PNF for cerebral palsy. Paper given at World Congress of World Confed. Phys. Ther. Amsterdam.

88 LEVITT S. (1969) The treatment of cerebral palsy and proprioceptive neuromuscular facilitation techniques, in *On the Treatment of Spastic Pareses.* Institute Neurology, Stockholm. *Sjukgymnasten* **27,** 3.

89 LEVITT S. (1967) Motor behaviour in cerebral palsy and relevant proprioceptive neuromuscular facilitation techniques. *Sjukgymnasten*, Nov. 1967 (from the Course given at Hindas, Sweden).

90 LEVITT S. (1966) Proprioceptive Neuromuscular Facilitation techniques in cerebral palsy. *Physiotherapy*, **52,** 46.

91 SCRUTTON D. & GILBERTSON M. (1975) *Physiotherapy in Paediatric Practice.* Butterworths, London.

92 FOLEY J. (1965) The treatment of cerebral palsy and allied disorders in the young child, in *Physical Medicine in Paediatrics*, ed. Kiernander B. Butterworths, London.

93 JOHNSTON & MAGRAB (1976) *Developmental Disorders: Assessment, Treatment, Education.* University Park Press, Baltimore.

94 GRENIER A. (1973) Small walking splint for cerebral palsy children. C.D.I. Cahiers. English edition, No. 2, Paris.

95 GRENIER A. (1973) Pes Valgoplanus in cerebral palsy. The therapeutic role of special shoes for cerebral palsy children. C.D.I. Cahiers. English Edition, No. 1.

96 NEUMANN NEURODDE D. (1967) *Baby Gymnastics.* Pergamon Press, London & Oxford.

97 KENDALL P. HUME (1961) Evaluation of treatment in cerebral palsy. *Dev. Med. Child Neurol.* **3,** (3), 495.

98 HOLT K.S. (1965) In *Assessment of Cerebral Palsy*, Chapter 1, Lloyd-Luke, London.

99 LEVITT S. (1957) Cerebral palsy. A critique of the evaluation of therapy. *Brit. J. Phys. Med.*, **20,** 6 (June).

100 WOLF J.M. (1969) (ed.) *The Results of Treatment in Cerebral Palsy;* particularly in *Part Four: Developmental and Assessment Scales.* C. C. Thomas, Springfield, Ill.

101 DURUKAN F. Ph.D. Thesis on Assessment in Cerebral Palsy at The Wolfson Centre, Institute of Child Health, University of London, 1977.

102 Analysis and Recording of Movement in Normal and Abnormal Subjects— A Workshop organised by B. J. Lewis, Anstey Dept. Physical Education, Birmingham Polytechnic *and* S. Levitt, The Wolfson Centre at the Institute of Child Health, London, May 1976 (in press).

103 HOLT K.S. (1975) (ed.) *Movement and Child Development.* Chapters 6, 7, 10, 11, 12. Heinemann—Spastics International Medical Publications, London.

104 HOLT K.S., JONES R.B. & WILSON R. (1974) Gait Analysis by means of a multiple sequential camera. *Dev. Med. Child Neurol,* **16,** 742.

105 HOLT K.S. (1973) Discussion of Equinus in Cahiers C.D.I. No. 1, English edn.

106 MORGENSTERN M., LOW-BEER H. & MORGENSTERN F. (1966) *Practical Training for the Severely Handicapped Child.* Heinemann, London.

107 BRERETON B. (1971) *Learning Ability.* The Spastics Centre, N.S.W., Australia.

108 BRERETON B. & SATTLER J. (1967) *Cerebral Palsy: Basic Abilities.* The Spastic Centre of New South Wales, Australia.

109 WHITING P.R. & MORRIS (1971) *Motor Impairment and Compensatory Education.* G. Bell, London.

110 CRATTY B. (1969) *Perceptuo-Motor Efficiency in Children.* Lea & Febiger, Philadelphia.

111 CRATTY B.J. (1967) *Developmental Sequence of Perceptuo-motor Tasks and Movement Activities for Neurologically Handicapped and Retarded Children.* New York Education Ach.

112 Consult literature in Special Education, Psychology, Occupational Therapy and Physical Education.

113 BURNS Y. (1970) Reduction of hypertonicity with the use of plasters. *Aust. J. Physiother,* **XVL,** 3 Sept.

114 DE RIJKE H., ALLEN D. CULLOTY V. & HARE N. (1965–1977) In demonstrations of plasters for children with spastic feet and other deformities, in cerebral palsy.

115 BREWER M. (1969) 'conducted' Nursery Group at Cheyne Walk Spastic Centre as first of the interdisciplinary groups at the Centre.

116 SEGLOW D. & COLLINS J. (1972) Pre-school help for children with cerebral palsy. Northern Ireland Region, 4 Annadale Ave, Belfast BT 7 2JH.

117 MILLER C.J. (1972) The Speech Therapist and the Group Treatment of Young Cerebral Palsied Children. *Brit. J. Dis. Com.* **7,** No. 2.

118 PARNWELL M. (1968) *The Integration of Disciplines.* Paper read The International Spastics Society Conference. Education Seminar, April. Oxford.

119 ZINKIN P. (1976) Visually handicapped Children's Clinics. The Wolfson Centre, Institute of Child Health, London.

INDEX